THE MEDICAL RECORD AS A FORENSIC RESOURCE

Campion Quinn, MD, MHA

JONES AND BARTLETT PUBLISHERS
Sudbury, Mass
BOSTON   TORONTO   L

D0274532

World Headquarters
Jones and Bartlett Publishers
40 Tall Pine Drive
Sudbury, MA 01776
978-443-5000
info@jbpub.com
www.jbpub.com

Jones and Bartlett Publishers Canada
2406 Nikanna Road
Mississauga, ON L5C 2W6
CANADA

Jones and Bartlett Publishers International
Barb House, Barb Mews
London W6 7PA
UK

Library of Congress Cataloging-in-Publication Data
Quinn, Campion.
   The medical record as a forensic resource / Campion Quinn.
      p. ; cm.
   Includes bibliographical references and index.
   ISBN 0-7637-2759-8 (pbk.)
      1. Medical records—Access control—United States. 2. Medical records—Law and legislation—United States. 3. Medical jurisprudence—United States.   I. Title.
      [DNLM: 1. Forms and Records Control—methods. 2. Forensic Medicine—methods.
   3. Medical Records—legislation & jurisprudence.   W 80 Q7m 2004]
   R864.Q55 2004
   614'.1—dc22

                                                          2004013530

Production Credits
Acquisitions Editor: Kevin Sullivan
Production Manager: Amy Rose
Associate Production Editor: Tracey Chapman
Editorial Assistant: Amy Sibley
Marketing Manager: Ed McKenna
Associate Marketing Manager: Emily Ekle
Manufacturing and Inventory Coordinator: Amy Bacus
Composition: Auburn Associates, Inc.
Cover Design: Kristin E. Ohlin
Printing and Binding: Malloy, Inc.
Cover Printing: Malloy, Inc.

Printed in the United States of America
08 07 06 05   10 9 8 7 6 5 4 3 2

Dedication

For my father, Edward Quinn,
who taught me everything important in life.

Table of Contents

Contributors

Karen A. Fielder, BSN, RN, JD, Esq.
Fumuso, Kelly, DeVerna, Snyder, Swart & Farrell, LLP

Edward L. Birnbaum
LLB Head of Litigation Department
Herzfeld & Rubin, PC

Carl T. Grasso, BS, JD
Herzfeld & Rubin, PC

Kimberly Zammit, PharmD, BCPS
Clinical Coordinator
Buffalo General Hospital

Acknowledgments

This book was vastly improved by the efforts of the contributors and reviewers.

Edward Birnbaum, Esq., and Carl Grasso, Esq., of the litigation department of the law firm Herzfeld and Rubin, PC, co-wrote Chapter 26, "The Medical Chart as Evidence."

Kimberly Zammit, Pharm.D., a clinical pharmacist at the Buffalo General Hospital, is the author of Chapter 25, "Medication Errors."

Karen Fielder, Esq., of the law firm Fumuso, Kelly, DeVerna, Snyder, Swart & Farrell, LLP, contributed Chapter 2, "Acquiring a Medical Record."

I'd also like to thank Edward Quinn; Manlio Loconte, MD; Nancy DiPilli, RN; Fran LaPiedra, RN; Maryann DiPilli, RN; and John Downing, Esq., for their review of the manuscript and many insightful suggestions.

Thanks to you all.

Introduction

An accurate interpretation of the medical chart is critical to the litigation of medical malpractice, personal injury, and product liability cases. However, medical records are filled with specialized vocabulary, obscure idioms, and unfamiliar abbreviations. The logic of even appropriate medical decisions can be hard to follow for the nonmedical reviewer. This makes the medical record difficult or impossible for a lawyer or other nonmedical professional to understand completely.

The Medical Record as a Forensic Resource is an attempt to bridge the gap of understanding between the legal world and the world of medicine. The book provides insight into the creation of a medical chart and explains what the chart says, what it doesn't say, and what it is supposed to say. The book allows the nonmedical reviewer to appreciate the contents of a medical chart, the purpose of the various notes, and the intent of the author of the note. Further, several chapters deal with topics such as the nature of personal injury, malpractice cases, the admissibility of the medical chart as evidence, and how to identify tampering with the medical chart.

This book offers examples, explanations, and checklists to aid the reviewer in the evaluation of the medical chart to prepare for a legal proceeding. It may also be used as a reference for others whose professional interests require an understanding of the medical chart. Likewise, health care professionals who deal with legal issues, such as legal nurse consultants, will find this book useful as a guide to the intersection of the legal and health care worlds.

CHAPTER 1

What Is the Medical Chart?

Q **What is the medical chart?**

A The medical chart can best be defined as a document that summarizes a patient's interaction with a physician or other health care provider. It is the principal repository of information concerning the patient's past medical care.

Q **Who is the author of the medical chart?**

A While the physicians and nurses who provide direct care to a patient may contribute the most to a chart, most medical personnel who interact with the patient, the patient's tissues, radiographs, or test results also add to the chart. These additional authors include, but are not limited to, pathologists, radiologists, psychiatrists, pharmacists, dietitians, social workers, and physical and occupational therapists.

Q **What is the purpose of the medical chart?**

A Modern physicians (like the author) are taught that the medical chart is a document whose sole purpose is the improvement of the patient's health. This is not true now, and perhaps it never has been.

The medical chart was originally used as an *aide memoir* for a physician; it recorded his previous treatments and future plans for a particular patient. The use of a medical note as a memory aid goes back to the oldest recorded physician notes. In fact, surviving papyri from pharaonic Egypt record notes containing patients' complaints and therapies used to cure them.

As medicine became more complex and groups of physicians began treating the same patient, the chart was used as both a memory aid and a means of communication between physicians.

Further changes occurred in the medical chart as time progressed. These changes were driven by parties both in- and outside of medicine. The goals of these parties were often at odds with one another, resulting in the confusion that is the modern medical chart.

The medical chart serves some of the following purposes:

- Communication
- Education
- Audit and Oversight
- Analysis and Synthesis

Communication

The role of the medical chart as a tool of communication is clear. The physician writes a note in the medical chart to himself or his colleagues who are caring for the same patient. When he returns to the chart, he can easily recall what has been done, and what is pending. The other physicians who read the chart can maintain the continuity of care without having to depend on the memory of the physician or patient, ensuring coordinated, rather than fragmented, delivery of treatment. The physician also communicates through the medical chart when he writes orders. With orders, the physician contacts many people in the hospital with requests, tests, consultants, therapies, and so on, for his patient.

Education

The medical chart can also act as an educational medium. When a physician writes an admission note, the resident, intern, and medical student learn about the patient, and also about the correct way to do a history and physical examination. They also learn how to synthesize data into a diagnosis and plan. When a specialist writes a consultation note, this helps the primary care physician understand the therapeutic approach to a disease state he or she may not be familiar with. When a surgeon describes surgical techniques and findings in an operative note, this helps the physicians to better understand the surgical technique, extent of disease, and potential disability.

Audit and Oversight

The medical chart is written for use not only by other physicians, but also for other interested parties. These parties include insurers, third party payers, public health officials, plaintiff's lawyers, hospital risk managers, and quality assurance personnel. For these parties, the chart exists to document professional work—to record what was done, by whom, to whom, when, where, why, and with what results and also to document diagnosis and assessment, treatment/services provided, and the patient's clinical course.

In a malpractice suit, the medical note can be the physician's best defense or the plaintiff's "Exhibit A." Malpractice defense firms and hospital risk managers encourage physicians to record every negative and positive finding, and every conversation with another physician, nurse, or family member. They encourage the physician to explore every issue mentioned by the patient and every differential diagnosis, no matter how fruitless it may seem. This type of burdensome documentation may prevent malpractice suits, but does nothing to improve patient care. In fact, it may, because it is so time consuming, detract from the length of interaction between the physician and the patient.

In order to provide risk management and malpractice protection, the physician and other health care personnel are required to provide the following documentation on a medical chart:

- All informed consents for treatments
- Any release of records, etc.
- Any professional decisions
- Any problems encountered in working with the patient
- Anything that will support the adequacy of the clinical assessment and the appropriateness of the treatment/service plan
- Any instance of the application of professional skills and knowledge in the provision of professional services
- Substantiation of the treatment/services provided and of the results of such treatment/services

In like manner, insurance companies use the medical chart to validate the billing requests. The physician is obligated to write a note that justifies the length and complexity of the exam. Finally, the medical chart is used to facilitate quality assurance and utilization review.

A quality assurance and utilization review has the following intentions:

- To record professional activities, their purposes, and results.
- To document the appropriateness, necessity, and effectiveness of treatment/services provided.
- To document the need for further treatment/services or to support termination of treatment/services.
- To facilitate supervision, consultation, and staff development.
- To help improve the quality of services by identifying problems with the delivery of service and providing data based upon which effective corrective action can be undertaken.
- To provide data for educational planning, policy development, program planning, and research.

Analysis and Synthesis of Information

The medical chart is also used as a place to collect data, to review the results for various tests, to examine possible diagnoses, and to synthesize a plan for further diagnostic tests or therapeutic options. Though this is the least appreciated use, it is perhaps the highest use of the medical chart by the physician and arguably the most important part of the chart for promoting patient health.

CHAPTER 2

Acquiring a Medical Record

Acquiring a medical record, for any purpose, can be a confusing and sometimes daunting task. This chapter will demystify that task by explaining the answers to the following questions:

- Who can request a medical record?
- Who can release the health information?
- To whom can the information be released?
- What information can be released?
- What are the implications of federal and state statutes and regulations that govern this process?

Who can request a medical record?

The medical record may legitimately be sought by many people, including physicians, attorneys, patients, public health workers, law enforcement officials, and health care insurers. These records are sought for many reasons including further treatment, medical research, litigation, and reimbursement issues. The key factor for any entity that is releasing a patient's information is to ensure that the medical record, or any other health information, is being released at the direction of a qualified person.

Who can release health information?

A "qualified person" is a legal term that is defined by a state or federal statute. A "qualified person" can be a patient, guardian appointed by law, parent of an infant, or representative acting on behalf of the patient's estate. When a representative acting on behalf of a patient's estate requests a medical record, he must attach with that request the appropriate Letters Testamentary (the legal document that gives the representative the authority to act on behalf of the estate).

Who owns the medical record?

Before health care information can be released, it is important to understand who owns the medical record and who owns the health care information. This entails identifying who owns the paper and who owns the information documented on that paper. Under most state laws, the medical record is the property of the entity that produced the document. However, state law typically provides that the health care information contained in the document is subject to the control of the patient.

Who can release health care information?

In most states, who can release or authorize release of medical records is governed by state law. In general, upon the written request of any competent patient, parent, or legal guardian, a health care provider or hospital must release and deliver copies of X-rays, medical records, and test results regarding the patient to any other designated party.[1] However, this does not include personal notes of the physician. The health care provider, or hospital, can charge a reasonable fee for photocopying. A qualified person—the patient—is entitled to inspect or photocopy his own records within a certain time frame provided he has made a written request to do so.

What is a reasonable fee for the medical records?

A health care provider or hospital may charge a reasonable fee for photocopying. This fee should not exceed what the actual cost is to the physician or hospital. However, it does not have to be solely based on the photocopying charges; it can include the cost of personnel to perform the task and any costs incurred in retrieving the medical record. Furthermore, the physician or hospital can request payment before photocopying or enclose a request for payment at a later date.

---

[1]NY PHL § 17 (McKinney's Supp.)

Q

A

**Can a physician or hospital
refuse to provide medical records?**

A physician or hospital that refuses to provide a qualified person with a copy or access to his or her medical record can be subject to a penalty. However, under certain circumstances a physician or hospital can withhold information. If a physician determines that release of certain information would be detrimental, and it could reasonably be expected to cause substantial and identifiable harm to the person, the information can be withheld.[2] Furthermore, sensitive materials, such as HIV/AIDS, psychiatric, and mental health records, are subject to further state confidentiality laws and require specific written authorization by the person before being released.

Q

A

How do you request the medical record?

The initial step in obtaining a medical record is to have the patient or qualified person sign an authorization. An authorization, or release of medical records, can come in many different forms. However, since the inception of the Health Insurance Portability and Accountability Act (HIPAA), several key factors must be included in the authorization.

Q

A

What is HIPAA?

The Health Insurance Portability and Accountability Act of 1996 is a federal law. The key purpose of the act was to put into place further safeguards to ensure confidentiality of patients' health care information. HIPAA protects all individually identifiable health information in any form—electronic, paper, or oral. The Act clearly states that protected health information cannot be disclosed without a valid authorization. So, to ensure compliance with the federal act, all authorizations must be HIPAA compliant.

Q

A

What must be contained within the authorization?

To be a HIPAA compliant authorization the language must be plain and simple. A lay person must easily understand it. The authorization must contain a specific description of the information to be disclosed, the identification of those authorized to disclose the information, the name of those to whom the infor-

---

[2] NY PHL § 18 (McKinney's Supp.)

mation may be disclosed, the purpose of the disclosure (or a statement indicating it is at the request of the individual), an expiration date, and a notarized signature and date from the individual. Furthermore, it must include a statement of the individual's right to revoke the authorization and a statement that information disclosed pursuant to the authorization may be subject to redisclosure and no longer protected by the rule.[3] Thus, if each of the elements is contained within the authorization, it is a valid authorization. (See Table 2.1.)

What specific information can be disclosed?

HIPAA requires that the specific information to be disclosed must be contained within an authorization and no other information be released. Thus, if you are a plaintiff in a personal injury action, then you will most likely want to limit what medical records are released to the defendant. This can be done by specifically identifying in the authorization what information you will allow to be released. For example, the authorization would clearly state what hospital and dates of admission and treatment could be released, thereby preventing the release of any other admissions to that hospital. However, if you are the defendant in that same action, you would want an authorization that provides for the release of any and all treatment at that hospital, including emergency department visits, outpatient clinic records, ambulatory surgery, and diagnostic testing.

Furthermore, any request for mental health or substance abuse records requires specific authorization to release. Before releasing any HIV/AIDS, mental health, or substance abuse medical records, specific authorization should be obtained. In addition, if medical records contain such information and the authorization does not specifically authorize the release of the same, this information should be redacted.

Is the provider releasing the health information identified in the authorization?

The authorization must identify who can release the information. The authorization must identify the health care provider, either physician or hospital, who is authorized to release the information. It should also contain the name and address of that party.

---

[3]http://www.hhs.gov/ocr/hipaa

Table 2.1   Example HIPAA Compliant Authorization

Patient Authorization for Disclosure of Protected Health Information

I, **(name)**, AUTHORIZE **(party releasing information)**, TO USE AND/OR DIS-CLOSE CERTAIN PROTECTED HEALTH INFORMATION ABOUT ME TO: **(name of party who information is to be released to)**

THIS AUTHORIZATION PERMITS THEM TO USE AND/OR DISCLOSE A COM-PLETE COPY OF YOUR RECORDS INCLUDING ALL INDIVIDUALLY IDENTIFIABLE HEALTH INFORMATION ABOUT ME. THE INFORMATION WILL BE USED OR DISCLOSED AT MY REQUEST.

THIS AUTHORIZATION WILL EXPIRE ON **(should not exceed 6 months)**

I HAVE THE RIGHT TO REFUSE TO SIGN THIS AUTHORIZATION. WHEN MY INFORMATION IS USED OR DISCLOSED PURSUANT TO THIS AUTHORIZATION, IT MAY BE SUBJECT TO RE-DISCLOSURE BY THE RECIPIENT AND MAY NO LONGER BE PROTECTED BY THE FEDERAL HIPAA PRIVACY RULE. I HAVE THE RIGHT TO REVOKE THIS AUTHORIZATION IN WRITING EXCEPT TO THE EXTENT THAT THE BEARER HAS ACTED IN RELIANCE UPON THIS AUTHORIZATION.

THIS AUTHORIZATION IS LIMITED TO THE FURNISHING OF THE BELOW DESCRIBED RECORDS ONLY. It is not to be construed as an authorization permit-ting you to disclose, orally or in writing, any of the additional information acquired by you in attending me in a professional capacity and which is not necessary to enable you to act in that capacity, nor does this authorization permit you to furnish anyone with any records, writings, conversations or other communications you may have had with my attorneys or their representatives.

❏ MEDICAL/ HOSPITAL record in your custody pertaining to the care and treat-ment of the above-named individual. MRN No:_____ Admission/Dates of Treatment_____

❏ NO-FAULT records relating to the accident of_____

❏ WORKERS' COMPENSATION/DISABILITY records relating to the accident on_____

❏ EMPLOYMENT/SCHOOL records for wage/attendance/grade information from _____to_____

❏ OTHER _____

_____
(signature)

On the   day of   , 20 , before me personally came and appeared the above named, to me known and known to me to be the individual described in and who executed the foregoing and who duly acknowledged to me that said per-son executed same.

NOTARY PUBLIC

Q   **Must the party who is receiving
the information be identified?**

A   The authorization must identify the party to whom the medical record is to be sent. Therefore, if multiple parties are to receive the same medical record, each and every party must have his or her own authorization that identifies him or her as the party receiving the medical record.

Q   **Does the purpose of the disclosure need to be identified?**

A   The authorization must contain a statement identifying the purpose of the authorization. For example, if the authorization is for health care reimbursement, then it should state that. In litigation, oftentimes the purpose will be stated as the request of the individual. This statement by the individual complies with the HIPAA requirements.

Q   **Does the authorization form have an expiration date?**

A   The authorization must contain an expiration date—a future date at which point the authorization is no longer valid. The expiration date should not exceed 6 months from the date the authorization is signed by the patient. This will ensure, for the patient, that only records up until a certain point in time are released. However, if you are the health care provider whose records are being sought, it is important, prior to releasing medical records, to check the expiration date. Releasing a medical record based on an authorization that has expired would be akin to releasing medical records without an authorization since the authorization is not valid.

Q   **Does the authorization need to
be signed, dated, and notarized?**

A   The authorization must contain the original notarized signature of the patient who is authorizing the release of the medical record. This is most important to the health care provider. The authorization should always be checked for an original signature. A notary public ensures the validity of that signature. This procedure protects the provider who is releasing the information by ensuring that the patient requesting the release of the information is the party that has signed the authorization.

It is only in a few circumstances when the authorization will be signed by someone other than the patient. These circumstances include when the patient is an infant (a minor) and the legal guardian or parent is authorizing the release of information, the patient has a guardian appointed by law, or the patient is deceased and the party representing the estate is authorizing release of information. In the latter two circumstances, additional documentation should accompany the authorization to ensure that those requesting the information do, in fact, have the legal authority to do so.

The date the patient signed the authorization should also be included. Again, this will ensure that the authorization is valid and provide a time frame to work within.

Q   **Can the information that has been disclosed be re-disclosed without a new authorization?**

A   A HIPAA compliant authorization includes a statement that makes it known to all parties (patient and health care provider) that the information may be subject to re-disclosure. Re-disclosed documents are no longer protected by the HIPAA guidelines. In litigation, this statement is very important. For example, defendants in a medical malpractice action may require expert opinions. An expert opinion is obtained by providing the expert witness with a complete copy of the medical record. Thus, the statement that the information may be re-disclosed is crucial since it informs the patient that others will be examining his or her medical record aside from the party they authorized.

Q   **How do you obtain a medical record?**

A   If you are the party seeking release of the medical record and you have a valid authorization, the next step is to forward, in the form of a letter, a request to the physician or hospital designated on the authorization. (See Table 2.2.)

Q   **What if the party does not respond?**

A   The party seeking the medical record should have a diary or calendar system to follow up on a request. A follow-up letter should be sent after a reasonable time if no response is received. A reasonable time can be anywhere from 2 weeks to 2 months.

Table 2.2   Letter of Request for a Medical Record

(Date)

(Name of Health Care Provider)
(Address)

Re: (Patient Medical Record) (D/O/B:)

Dear Sir or Madam:

Please be advised that this office is authorized by the above-named patient to obtain a complete copy of the patient's medical record.

Kindly furnish us with a copy of your <u>complete office records as well as your billing records in connection with the above-named patient. An authorization signed by the patient permitting the release of this information is enclosed.</u>

Additionally, should there be a fee for a copy of the medical record, please provide an invoice for the reasonable cost therein.

It would be greatly appreciated if you could expedite this request. Should you have any questions, please do not hesitate to contact the undersigned. Thank you for your prompt attention to this matter.

Very truly yours,

(Signature)
(Name)

If the provider still does not comply with the patient's request for medical records, a reason for the provider's refusal should be sought. In some rare instances, the provider can deny access if it is believed that the information contained within the medical record will cause substantial harm to the patient. These are very limited situations and governed by state law. Otherwise, a provider's failure to comply with a patient's duly authorized request for medical records can result in legal sanctions.

Q   Are there other ways to obtain a medical record?

A   There are other ways to obtain a patient's medical record including a court order and a *subpoena duces tecum*.

general description of who the recipients of the information will be
the date and signature of patient

What should be asked about the authorization for release of information?

Have unauthorized people seen the information?
Who signed the authorization?
If the patient signed the authorization, was the patient competent to give authorization?
If a proxy for the patient signed the authorization, was the
proxy empowered to give authorization by statute or legal
instrumentality (i.e., power-of-attorney form, health care
proxy, or living will)?
If a proxy signed the authorization, is the legal instrument
that empowers the proxy still in force?
Does the legal instrument need to be updated, that is, has
the patient's condition substantially improved or become
hopeless?
Have the wishes of the patient changed?

- A *court order* is a directive from a judge. The court can order
  a witness to produce a patient's medical record. If the court
  order is signed by a judge, failure to comply with the court's
  directive could result in sanctions.
- A *subpoena duces tecum* is a command to a witness to produce documents. A *subpoena duces tecum* may be issued
  without a court order. In the area of personal injury, it is
  often used to obtain medical records. The subpoena can be
  issued by an attorney for a party in a lawsuit. However, individual states have started to require that an authorization
  from the patient accompany the subpoena. It would be wise
  to seek legal advice prior to releasing medical records pursuant to a *subpoena duces tecum*, especially since, for the
  release of mental health or other highly sensitive material, a
  court order is also required to accompany the subpoena.

CONCLUSION

The process of acquiring the medical record can be difficult at times.
However, diligence and close attention to detail will accomplish the goal.
Special attention to the authorization in the initial stage will avoid problems and delays. Check the authorization for the key requirements (such
as appropriate signature, dates, notarization, HIPAA requirements, etc.)
before forwarding to the health care provider. Checking the authorization
for the very same requirements before releasing records enables both
sides to be as expeditious as possible.

- A
  ti
- T

Q   wl
     au

     -
     -
     -
     -

     -

Authorization for
of Medical Inforn

Q   **What is the authorization for
     release of medical information?**

A   The authorization for release of m(
     cialized consent form. When signed,
     rizes the physician, hospital, or othe
     the patient's medical information t(
     These interested entities can include
     insurance companies, third party adn
     nance organizations, and the health d(

Q   **Who creates the authorization for
     release of medical information form?**

A   The authorization form is produced by
     (or his guardian) is the signatory.

Q   **What does the authorization
     for release of information contain?**

A   The authorization document contains the

     - An explanation of the purpose of the d
       process insurance claims and comply v
       public health law)
     - A general description of what informati(

CHAPTER 4

Determining What Is Missing from a Medical Chart

When an attorney requests a medical chart from a physician, clinic, or hospital, it is often assumed that a copy of the complete chart will be sent. In the author's experience, this rarely happens. Often parts of the medical chart may be missing due to misfiling, incompetence, or malfeasance.

Q **How do you determine what is missing from the medical chart?**

A Before starting the formal chart review, the following should be done in order to ensure that a complete copy is available for review:

- When the copy of the chart is received, review it with a checklist (see Appendix 3), making sure that all the requested items have been received.
- After the chart has been organized categorically and chronologically, the reviewer should cross-reference the information and ask the following questions:
  - Does the ED chart refer to an ambulance report that is not present?
  - Do the surgeon's notes refer to pre-operative testing that is not in the chart?
  - Do all physician orders for consultations have corresponding consultant's reports?

- Do all physician orders for laboratory and radiology tests have the corresponding lab and X-ray reports?
- Do all physician orders for medication have nurse medication administration records?
- Are all consultants' requests for action (e.g., medications, diagnostic tests, surgery, and other medical or surgical consultations) recorded in the physician order forms as well as in the physician and nurse records?
- Do all requests for physician evaluation or assistance found in nursing notes have corresponding action notes in the physician record?
- Do all notations of incidents and adverse events mentioned in the nursing notes have a corresponding note in the physician record?
- Do all reports of tests, radiographs, surgeries, and therapies mentioned in the discharge note correspond with the events reported in the medical chart?
- Do all biopsies include surgical procedure notes?

- Other questions to ask:
  - Are ambulance call reports, transfer notes, or pre-admission testing records included in the hospital report?
  - Were any reports developed subsequent to the patient's discharge that do not appear in the current medical record (e.g., laboratory results, dictated procedure notes, and autopsy reports)?
  - Should the records from preceding or subsequent hospitalizations be requested?
  - Should the records from outpatient clinics or private physician offices be requested?
  - Should the pharmacy records from the hospital or outpatient pharmacy be requested?
  - Did the patient have follow-up treatments?
  - Should all the records for follow-up treatments be requested?
  - Should I have records for the patient's admissions to other facilities as a result of occurrences during the hospitalization in question?
  - Did other physicians treat the patient before or after the incident in question? Should I have these physicians' office records?

- Does the physician's office record contain all of the physician's notes, consultant's notes, and laboratory and X-ray reports?
- Do the physician's office notes contain reports on phone conversations with the patient or family? Are these stored somewhere else?
- Should a copy of the ED or clinic log be requested? Sometimes a defendant alleges that the clinic or ED was so busy that it was impossible to render adequate care to a particular patient. Information regarding how many patients were actually there can substantiate this claim.
- Should a copy of the physician or nurse's schedule be requested? When it is difficult to read signatures or initials on a chart, having a copy of the names of the individuals on duty at the time can be very helpful. Further, if there were too few nurses or physicians scheduled to be on duty to treat the patients, the hospital could be held liable for creating an unsafe environment.

Q
A

How to get what's missing from the chart?

When it is determined that the medical chart is incomplete, a list of the missing sections should be made. This list should be as explicit as possible, including dates of tests, names of consultants, types of surgical procedures, and so on. This list of missing elements should be forwarded to the attorney so that a complete medical record can be requested and secured.

CHAPTER 5

How to Examine an Individual Medical Chart

Once the medical chart has been delivered, the reviewer is responsible for developing an analysis and summary of the chart to aid legal counsel in defense or prosecution of the case. In order to create this analysis and summary, the medical reviewer must complete the following tasks:

- Determine if the entire medical record is present
- Organize the medical record categorically and chronologically
- Perform an analysis of the information
- Create tables, illustrations, and time lines
- Render an opinion

Q **Can you have too much medical information or too many medical records?**

A The answer to this important question is a definite yes. If the negligence case revolves around a single incident, say a surgical misadventure or a patient falling out of bed, acquiring many years of medical records will not aid the reviewer in rendering an opinion. In fact, too many records could tend to obfuscate the event. If, however, the causation of an injury or illness is unclear, a lengthy review of all available medical records may help to determine the cause. If the causation of the tort is known before the medical record is requested, then the review can be limited to those medical reports occurring just before and just after the incident. However, if the causation is unknown, it is better to request more information than less.

Q   **What can you do if the copies of the medical record are of poor quality or the writing is illegible?**

A   If the copy is too poor to read (e.g., too light, off-centered, or covered by another document), the plaintiff can request a better copy. This request should be forwarded to the attorney. If the handwriting in a particular note is illegible, the note should be copied and forwarded to the attorney. This note will then be reviewed with the author at a deposition.

Q   **What do you do when you have a completed medical chart?**

A   When the entire medical chart is available, the reviewer should complete the following tasks:

- Take the chart apart.
- Arrange the chart into groups of "like reports" (e.g., physician progress notes, radiology reports, rehab notes, physician's orders, and nursing progress notes).
- Take each group of "like reports" and arrange them in chronological order.
- Place these ordered pages together in one group.
- Number each page. Numbering stamps are inexpensive and are readily available in most office product stores. The page number should be in the same place on each page. Page numbers allow reviewers and attorneys to reference the material easily.
- Make at least three copies of complete medical record on pre-drilled three-hole paper. (The reviewer should be careful to keep the original copy intact, as hole punching sometimes destroys vital information.)
  - Place each copy of the chart into a three-ring binder. Each group of "like reports" should be separated with page dividers and labeled with tabs.
  - Copy 1 should be designated as the consultant's copy. This chart should not be marked or highlighted in any way.
  - Copy 2 should be designated as the working copy. In this chart, the reviewer and legal team are free to underline, flag, highlight, and make marginal notes.
  - Copy 3 should be held in reserve for unexpected contingencies, such as a lost copy, the need for a second consultant copy, or a copy for another attorney.

Q
A

What do you do when the chart is complete and organized?

Once the chart has been reviewed several times, the reviewer can create a summary. A summary accomplishes several goals for the attorney. It spares the attorney the need to read through voluminous medical records of questionable probative value. It focuses on the important events recorded, and it interprets medical jargon and concepts that may be difficult for nonmedical personnel to understand.

Q
A

What is a summary document?

The summary document should include the following information:

- Date of patient's admission or date when the physician-patient relationship began.
- Names of treating physicians and their qualifications. *A physician's training and board certification can be confirmed by checking with the American Medical Association or with the local medical or specialty society.*
- Times and dates of significant medical findings (e.g., new diagnoses, lab test results, new fevers, and a drop in blood pressure).
- Times and dates of significant medical events (e.g., cardiac arrest, trip and fall, allergic reaction, and drug misadministration).
- Times and dates of significant medical tests (e.g., CT scans, MRIs, EKGs, and blood tests)
- Times and dates of significant statements by the patient. *These statements are often recorded by the ambulance crew, ED staff, and physicians writing the admission note. These spontaneous utterances are considered to have great probative value, since they are made before the patient has had time to reflect on issues of negligence or monetary recovery.*
- Times and dates of significant statements, requests, or orders by physicians or nurses.
- Copies of any photos taken of the patient's wounds, disabilities, or disfigurements. *These photographs should be captioned and dated.*
- Medical Illustrations of relevant anatomy, wounds, burn areas, surgical procedures, etc. *These illustrations should be simplified and clearly demonstrate the medical issue at hand. Overly*

complex diagrams or poorly captioned illustrations will not achieve the clarity the reviewer is seeking. These illustrations can be created by a local artist, copied from textbooks, or created using medical illustration software. These illustrations should be stored as digital files. In digital format, the illustration can be easily enlarged if it needs to be used as a courtroom exhibit.

- Charts and tables. *Charts and tables are an excellent way to compare changes to sets of facts. A table is a graphic layout of columns and rows of boxes. Each box contains a set of information that is compared with the other boxes along the horizontal axis. For example, the ideal therapeutic approach to a patient is compared (in the next column) to the approach used by the physician under scrutiny. Alternatively, one column could contain abilities of the patient before the accident; the next column could contain the patient's altered abilities after the accident. (See Table 5.1.)*

Table 5.1   A Comparative Table

Approaches to a Patient with Chest Pain	
American College of Cardiologists' Recommendations for Evaluation of Chest Pain	Dr. Smith's Approach to the Evaluation of Chest Pain
Interview patient	Interview patient
Perform physical examination	Perform physical examination
Perform and interpret ECG	CT of abdomen
Draw blood for cardiac enzymes	Draw blood for CBC and blood cultures
Insert intravenous line of normal saline	Consult surgery
Place on cardiac monitor	Admit to surgical unit
Administer nitrates	
Administer nasal O_2	
Consult cardiology	
Perform chest X-ray	
Repeat ECG and cardiac enzymes	
Admit to cardiac care unit	

- Time line of events. *The time line is a quick way of demon-strating a complex sequence of events, such as the course of a hospitalization or events leading up to and following a particular procedure. The time line consists of a horizontal line, which represents the passage of time. Along the horizontal line, "event boxes" are attached in accord with their chronological occurrence. The event boxes are filled with the brief abstract of the events outlined in the case summary. These abstracts are placed in the "event boxes" and then are attached to a horizontal line in accord with their chronology. (See Tables 5.2 and 5.3.)*

Table 5.2   Time Line 1

Time Line
Evaluation of John Doe's Mole

05/15/03	JD enters Dr. Jones's office and complains of mole on back. Dr. Jones reports that it is a benign mole and has the patient follow up in six months.
11/02/03	JD returns to Dr. Jones's office. He states the mole has been "bleeding," and he wants it biopsied. Dr. Jones reexamines the mole. Dr. Jones states that the mole is benign, and he sees no bleeding. Dr. Jones tells the patient to return in six months.
03/10/04	JD enters the office of Dr. Smith, an internist. Dr. Smith examines JD's mole. Dr. Smith states the mole looks "scary" and recommends a biopsy with a wide excision.
03/14/04	JD returns to Dr. Jones's office and asks for a referral to a surgeon for a biopsy. Dr. Jones reexamines the mole and discusses why he thinks that the mole is benign. He asks the patient to return in six months for a reevaluation.
06/02/04	JD returns to Dr. Jones's office. He states that his wife has noticed the mole is larger, and it is bleeding more frequently. Dr. Jones examines the mole and refers JD to a dermatologist.
07/14/04	JD is examined by Dr. Forte, a dermatologist. Dr. Forte states that the mole appears to be a melanoma and recommends immediate biopsy.
07/20/04	JD has biopsy of mole performed by Dr. Dinny, a general surgeon.
07/25/04	The mole is diagnosed pathologically as melanoma.
07/28/04	JD undergoes chest X-ray and CT scan of head. These reveal widely metastasized melanoma.
08/15/04	JD begins chemotherapy.

continues

Table 5.2   (continued)

Time Line
Evaluation of John Doe's Mole

11/18/04	Repeat CT reveals increased metastasis.
12/03/04	JD expires in ICU of General Hospital from expanding brain tumor.

Table 5.3   Time Line 2

Time Line

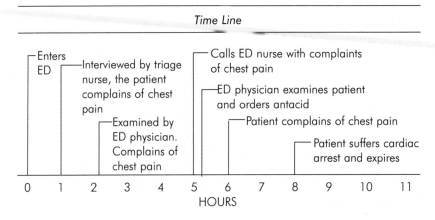

- Assessment. *The assessment should include answers to the following questions:*
  - What is the final diagnosis?
  - What is the proximate cause of the injury or illness?
  - Are these injuries mild, moderate, or severe?
  - Does the patient have any disabilities as a result of this accident or illness?
  - How disabled is the patient now? *Is it minimal, partial, or complete? Be as specific as possible. Mention how this disability will affect not only his employment, but also his ability to enjoy life.*
  - Are these disabilities or disfigurements temporary or permanent?
  - What are the likely future medical needs of the patient?
  - Is this condition likely to improve, or can the patient expect worsening illness or disability?

CHAPTER 6

Face Sheet

Q

A

What is the face sheet?

The face sheet is a document created at the time of admission. It contains demographic and financial documentation for the hospital's use.

Q

A

Who creates the face sheet?

The face sheet is usually created by the registrar at the hospital's admission office. In the case of emergencies, the face sheet may be filled out by the ED registrar or nurses.

Q

A

What does the face sheet contain?

The face sheet contains the following basic patient information:

- Patient name
- Date of birth
- Address
- Phone number
- Name and phone number of next of kin
- Religion
- Social security number
- Medical record number
- Insurance information

- Name of responsible party
- Date of admission

Q

What should be asked about the face sheet?

A

Confirm the patient's demographic data with other sources of information.

- Is the address the same? *The address, in addition to being an identifying element, can be a factor in the venue of litigation. If the patient uses a relative's address, rather than his or her own, to bring an action in a more "paternalistic" jurisdiction, the correct address on the hospital chart would serve as a basis for a change of venue to the legally appropriate jurisdiction.*
- Are the social security numbers the same? *It is necessary to find a match in the indices of claimant records, hospital records, insurance, motor vehicle, and bureau of criminal investigation (BCI) scan records.*
- Is the date of admission the same as the date of accident? If not, why not? *The date of admission is another significant element of validation. The date and time of hospital admission must be in sync with the claimed cause of the admission and treatment. The date and time of omission must be manifestly "post event," but in proximity to the claimed onset of a significant pathology or injury that is treated later. A failure to seek immediate treatment may suggest an intervening cause of injury, as would a documented diagnosis or treatment before the claimed incipient event. A situation where a laborer who injures his leg playing football is treated at the ED and then complains of leg pain on the job site is a skeletal outline of a possible deception.*
- Is the date of birth the same? *The date of birth is a significant date to confirm. It is likely to be more accurate than other sources as it must be consistent with insurance credentials. It has been noted that "scammers" often disguise their date of birth by using the wrong year or by scrambling the sequence of digits, so the motor vehicle bureau, criminal, and court records cannot be accessed easily. The scrambling of digits allows the scammer to make a plausible denial of fraudulent intent by maintaining the error in birth dates as a typo or misinterpretation.*

- Was the insurance information correct? *Insurance information tells the investigator how the hospital and medical bills are being paid, and, many times, what entity the patient believes should be responsible for payment (for example, the designation of the compensation carrier would be indicative of a perception of a work-related accident; a no fault carrier would suggest that incipient cause was an automobile accident). Some resourceful, unscrupulous patients, fashion the facts to suit the most favorable forum for recovery.*
- What is the name and phone number of next of kin? *The name and phone number of next of kin can be insightful for comparison with other legal or quasi-legal representations, such as insurance beneficiary claims for loss of consortium, location of witnesses, etc.*
- Who is the responsible party? *The responsible party is a person or entity who is not the insured or the patient but has financial responsibility for the patient's medical debts (often an employer). The designation of the responsible party may suggest a differing relationship than one indicated in the course of a litigation. The plaintiff may claim to be impoverished or indigent but may, in fact, identify an employer who compensates him or her regularly, or even handsomely. Alternatively, when a plaintiff claims to be a widow, divorced, or disabled, she may contradict those representations in her designation of her spouse or employer as the responsible party.*

CHAPTER 7

Consent Forms

Q

What is informed consent?

A

Informed consent is a person's agreement to allow something to happen (such as surgery). This consent should be based on a full disclosure of the facts needed to make the decision intelligently. In medicine, as in most other venues, every individual of adult years and sound mind has the right to determine what shall be done with his or her own body and control the course of his or her own medical treatment.[1] That is, a patient has a legal right to informed consent.

Q

What are the requirements of full disclosure?

A

When obtaining consent for a procedure, treatment, or medical, surgical, or psychological intervention, the medical provider should disclose the following information:

- The projected or desired outcomes of the proposed treatment and the likelihood of success
- Reasonably foreseeable risks or hazards inherent in the proposed treatment or care (this must be done in a manner that the patient can understand)

---

[1]Schoendorff v. Society of New York Hospital.

- Alternatives to proposed care or treatment plan
- Consequences of forgoing the treatment

Is informed consent necessary?

Informed consent is required by law and is derived from the theory that performing a procedure or treatment on a patient, without full disclosure of risks and benefits and the patient's informed consent, constitutes battery.

Below are criteria for obtaining informed consent:

- The patient must consent voluntarily.
- The patient must have the capacity to give consent.
- The patient must be an adult (under existing state law).
- In the event that the patient is a minor, or adult without capacity to consent, parents, attorneys, or legal guardians must give consent.
- The patient must have a full understanding of the scope of the intervention with all its attendant risks, benefits, and alternatives.
- The medical provider must obtain informed consent prior to the intervention.
- The medical provider must document the consent. *A signed consent agreement is adequate.*

Is there more than one type of consent form?

Before being treated, the patient must sign consent forms for both "routine care" and "nonroutine care." *Routine care* consists of standard, low-risk procedures, such as the administration of medications, phlebotomy, the insertion of intravenous lines, and routine diagnostic tests such as X-rays and ultrasound exams. *Nonroutine care* consent forms are for surgical procedures or other diagnostic or therapeutic interventions that have a higher risk.

What is contained in a consent form?

The following information is contained in the consent form:

- Date of consent
- Date of procedure
- Name and description of procedure

- Attestation that the risks and benefits of the proposed procedure were explained to the patient or guardian
- Signature of patient or guardian
- Signature of person asking for consent
- Signature of witness to consent

Q **What should be asked about consent forms?**

- Are the consent forms signed by the patient or legal guardian?
- Are the consent forms dated before the start of treatment?
- Was the patient able or competent enough to give informed consent at the time?
- Was the patient suffering great physical pain during the consent process?
- Had the patient suffered a head injury before giving consent?
- Had the patient received narcotics or sedatives that may have clouded his judgment?
- Was the patient intoxicated (i.e., under the influence of drugs, alcohol, or another toxic substance) while giving consent?
- Do the consent forms clearly describe the procedures as well as the risks and benefits of undergoing them?
- Was the consent form co-signed by the physician who performed the procedure? Or was it an intern, medical student, or nurse?
- Was the co-signer of the consent form able (knowledgeable) enough to explain all the risks and benefits to the patient?

CHAPTER **8**

Living Will/Power of Attorney

The federal Patient Self-Determination Act requires that all patients admitted to a hospital be informed about advance directives. Though they are encouraged to do so, patients are not required to execute these instruments. When these documents are signed and entered into the medical chart, the implementation of these directives is enforced by state law. State law allows the patients to leave very specific instructions for the health care team. In many states, for example, a patient may refuse cardiac and respiratory intervention but not refuse nutrition and/or hydration.

 What is a living will? (See Figure 8.1.)

 The *living will* (also known as a medical directive or advance directive) is a written document that records a person's wishes regarding life support or other medical treatments under certain circumstances. The living will transfers decision-making ability to another person when the patient is no longer competent to make decisions on his or her own behalf.

Q **What is a power of attorney? (See Figure 8.2.)**

A A *power of attorney* is a written instrument authorizing a person, the attorney-in-fact, to act as agent for another person to the extent indicated in the instrument.

LIVING WILL OF John Doe

I, John Doe, a resident of the City of Brooklyn, County of Kings, State of New York, being of sound and disposing mind, memory and under-standing, do hereby willfully and voluntarily make, publish and declare this to be my LIVING WILL, making known my desire that my life shall not be artificially prolonged under the circumstances set forth below, and do hereby declare:

1. This instrument is directed to my family, my physician(s), my attorney, my clergyman, any medical facility in whose care I happen to be, and to any individual who may become responsible for my health, welfare or affairs.
2. Let this statement stand as an expression of my wishes now that I am still of sound mind, for the time when I may no longer take part in decisions for my own future.
3. If at any time I should have a terminal condition and my attending physician has determined that there can be no recovery from such condition and my death is imminent, where the application of life-prolonging procedures and "heroic measures" would serve only to artificially prolong the dying process, I direct that such procedures be withheld or withdrawn, and that I be permitted to die naturally. For the sake of clarity, I do not wish to undergo the following life-prolonging procedures in the case of a hopeless diagnosis: artificial respiration, ventilators, hyperalimentation, feeding tubes (naso-gastric and percu-taneous), chemotherapy or radiation therapy. It is my intention to be spared the indignities of deterioration, dependence and hopeless pain. I therefore ask that medication be mercifully administered to me and that any medical procedures be performed on me that are deemed necessary to provide me with comfort, care or to alleviate pain.
4. In the absence of my ability to give directions regarding the use of such life-prolonging procedures, it is my intention that this declaration shall be honored by my family and physician as the final expression of my legal right to refuse medical or surgical treatment. I accept the consequences for such refusal.
5. In the event that I am diagnosed as comatose, incompetent, or oth-erwise mentally or physically incapable of communication, I appoint Jane Doe (my wife) to make binding decisions concerning my medi-cal treatment.

Figure 8.1   Living Will

6. I understand the full import of this declaration and I am emotionally and mentally competent to make this declaration that is based on my firmly held convictions.

IN WITNESS WHEREOF, I have hereunto subscribed my name and affixed my seal at _____, _____, this _____ day of _____, 20____, in the presence of the subscribing witnesses whom I have requested to become attesting witnesses hereto.

_____
Declarant

The declarant is known to me and I believe him/her to be of sound mind.

_____   _____
Witness   Address

NEW YORK HEALTH CARE PROXY/
Power of Attorney
(New York Public Health Law, Article 29-C, Section 2981)

I, (name of principal)

_____

hereby appoint: (name, home address and telephone number of agent)

_____

_____

as my health care agent to make any and all health care decisions for me, except to the extent I state otherwise. This health care proxy shall take effect in the event I become unable to make my own health care decisions.

NOTE: Although not necessary, and neither encouraged nor discouraged, you may wish to state instructions or wishes, and limit your agent's authority.

continues

Figure 8.2   New York Health Care Proxy

Figure 8.2   continued

Unless your agent knows your wishes about artificial nutrition and hydration, your agent will not have authority to decide about artificial nutrition and hydration. If you choose to state instructions, wishes, or limits, please do so below:

_____

_____

_____

_____

I direct my agent to make health care decisions in accordance with my wishes and instructions as stated above or as otherwise known to him or her. I also direct my agent to abide by any limitations on his or her authority as stated above or as otherwise known to him or her. In the event the person I appoint above is unable, unwilling or unavailable to act as my health care agent, I hereby appoint (name, home address and telephone number of alternate agent)

_____

_____

_____

as my health care agent.

I understand that, unless I revoke it, this proxy will remain in effect indefinitely or until the date or occurrence of the condition I have stated below:

(Please complete the following if you do NOT want this health care proxy to be in effect indefinitely):

This proxy shall expire: _____ (Specify date or condition)

Signature:

_____

Address:

_____

_____

Date:

_____

I declare that the person who signed or asked another to sign this document is personally known to me and appears to be of sound mind and acting willingly and free from duress. He or she signed (or asked another to sign for him or her) this document in my presence and that person signed in my presence. I am not the person appointed as agent by this document.

Witness:

_____

Address:

_____

_____

Witness:

_____

Address:

_____

_____

Q　**What should be asked about these instruments?**

- What do the advanced directives state about resuscitation, intravenous lines, feeding tubes, and so on?
- When was the document executed?
- Is the document still in force?
- Are any of the directives contradictory in their intent? (for example, the instrument stipulates no use of O_2 but *requests full resuscitation efforts to be made in case of respiratory failure*).
- Were the advanced directives entered into the physician's notes and orders?
- Was the person who gave direction to the physician regarding medical therapies the person named in the living will or power of attorney?

CHAPTER 9

Preadmission Records

Q
A
What are preadmission records?

Preadmission records are common documents found in the medical charts of elective hospital or surgical center admissions. An *elective admission* is a scheduled hospitalization for a planned procedure or therapy (e.g., surgery, blood transfusion, labor, and delivery). The *preadmission records* are medical documents that attest to the suitability of the patient to undergo a particular surgery or other therapy.

Q
A
Who is the author of the preadmission record?

The preadmission record may have many authors depending on what it contains. Typical authors are internists, family physicians, cardiologists, pulmonologists, pathologists, and radiologists.

Q
A
What does the preadmission record contain? (See Figure 9.1.)

At its most basic, a preadmission record contains a medical report (often from a primary care physician) that describes a medical history, physical examination, basic laboratory and radiology studies, and a statement to the effect that the surgery does not present an excessive risk to the patient.

The preadmission record can also include the following information:

St. Joseph's Hospital
Pre-Admission Testing Form

Last Name:	First Name:	Middle Initial:	Sex: M or F
Street Address:	City:	State:	ZIP code:
SS#:	Employer's Name:	Employer's Address:	
Name of Insured:		Relation to Insured:	
Insurance Company Name:	Insurance Group #:	Name of Primary Physician:	Primary Physician's Phone #:

Proposed Surgical Procedure:

Names of Current Medications:

Medical History:

Results of Physical Exam:

Lab Results:

Chest X-ray:	CBC:	PT/PTT:	ECG (attach original ECG to this form)
SMA—6:	Urinalysis:	Pulmonary Function Tests:	Echocardiogram:

Clinical Impression:

Is this patient medically stable to undergo the proposed anesthesia and the surgical procedure?

Examining Physician's Name:	Examining Physician's Signature:	Examining Physician's Phone #:	Date of this report:

Figure 9.1   Preadmission Testing Form

- Specialist consultation (cardiologist, pulmonologist, hematologist, or nephrologist)
- Blood tests
- Complete blood count
- Electrocardiogram
- Pulmonary function tests
- Chest X-ray
- CT scan
- MRI scan

Q **What should be asked about preadmission records?**

- Was a medical clearance given before surgery?
- Who gave the medical clearance for the procedure?
- Was the medical doctor qualified by training or experience to give a medical clearance for a surgical procedure?
- Are preadmission records complete? *In other words, are any standard tests missing?*
- Are any tests referred to in subsequent medical records that don't appear in the preadmission records?
- Were appropriate tests ordered?
- Were there foreseeable risks to surgery or anesthesia?
- Were there underlying diseases recorded that needed to be explored further? *Were there cardiac, hepatic, or metabolic diseases? Were there bleeding tendencies? Were their existing infections?*
- Were there chronic diseases that resulted in dysfunction that needed to be assessed?
- Were the tests completed near enough to the surgery to be meaningful?
- Were any abnormalities discovered that should have resulted in a cancellation of surgery but didn't?
- Is there any indication that the results were sent to the surgeon or treating physician before the procedure?
- Is there any indication in the notes that the surgeon or treating physician read the preadmission record (e.g., a signature on the forms or a dictated note)?

CHAPTER 10

Ambulance Call Report

What is the ambulance call report?

The ACR, or ambulance call report, is a report of the activities of the ambulance crew as they relate to their interaction with a specific patient. The ACR is also referred to as the emergency medical technician (EMT) record, the ambulance medical record, or field medical report. Because of the nature of the medical situation (emergent) and the qualifications of the medical providers (mid-level practitioners), the ACR tends to be short and the comments and descriptions terse. There is, however, a large amount of information to be found in this record, and it bears careful reading.

Who develops the ambulance call report?

The ACR is produced by one or more members of the ambulance crew. When reading ACRs, it is important to recall that all ambulance crews are not the same, nor are all members of a specific crew equally qualified. Some ambulance services are paid by a hospital or municipality and their crews can be well trained and highly skilled. Other ambulance services may be staffed by volunteers with little or no training or experience. Typically, an ambulance crew includes a driver and one or two medical technicians who care for the patient. The crew may include trained medical personnel such as EMTs, nurses, or relatively unskilled personnel with minimum training and little or no experience.

While a physician is rarely in the ambulance with the crew, physicians may arrive at the scene of illness or accident as "good samaritans." Further, some ambulance crews are in contact with their receiving hospital, and they may solicit medical advice from ED physicians via radio or cell phone. These physicians' comments or instructions may be recorded on the ACR.

Q

A

What is included in the ambulance call report?

The following information is typically included in the ACR:

- Name of person writing the note
- Names of ambulance crew members
- Badge numbers of the crew
- Time of notification of emergency
- Time of arrival at scene
- Time of departure from scene
- Time of arrival at ED, clinic, or hospital
- Location of accident
- Location of patient at the accident scene
- Name of patient
- Patient demographics (i.e., age, date of birth, address, next of kin, etc.)
- Chief complaint of patient or witnesses
- History of current illness
- Patient medical history
- Allergies
- Vital signs
- Brief physical examination
- Consultation with physicians/ED
- Treatments/procedures done in the field or ambulance
- Medications given
- Restraints, splints, or MAST trousers used
- Name of receiving hospital
- Name of physician accepting patient

Q

What should be asked about the ACR?

- Who wrote the ACR?
- Who was on the ambulance crew at the time of the call?
- What type of training or certification do the members of the

crew have (e.g., CPR, ACLS, ATLS, or basic life support [BLS])? *When evaluating an ambulance record, it is important to determine who is writing the note, their level of training, and length of experience. This information speaks to their level of ability and responsibility in caring for and treating the patient. It also suggests how much credibility can be given to the author's clinical observations.*

- What time was the ambulance notified?
- How long did it take the ambulance to respond to the scene?
- Was the response time appropriate?
- Were there inappropriate delays in transfer?
- How long was the ambulance at the scene?
- Did they spend too much time evaluating and treating the patient in the field when transfer to the ED for definitive diagnosis and treatment was indicated? *The various transfer times as well as the amount of time at the scene should be calculated. An estimate of the mileage and optimum transfer times should be compared with the recorded transfer times. Dramatic differences between expected and observed times should be explained by the ambulance crew. Prolonged time spent at the scene should be explained.*
- How did the crew describe the scene of the accident?
- What was the location of the patient when the ambulance arrived?
- Did the patient move himself, or was the patient moved from the original scene of the accident?
- If someone moved the patient, what was his or her name and relationship to the patient? *The exact location of the accident has a significant impact on the liability in personal injury cases. Variation of just a few feet can affect the status of the defendant. The reviewer should carefully note the location of the accident or of the patient that is mentioned by the ambulance crew.*
- What was the patient's condition on arrival of the ambulance?
- Did the patient's condition improve or deteriorate en route to the hospital?
- What medical interventions did the ambulance crew attempt or accomplish during their contact with the patient (e.g., medications, cardiopulmonary resuscitation (CPR), intravenous fluids, bandages, and restraints)?
- Did the patient ever stop breathing or lose his or her blood pressure?
- Did the patient receive an intravenous line? Why?

- What intravenous solution was administered to the patient (e.g., normal saline, Ringer's lactate, or dextrose 10%)?
- How much intravenous fluid was given in the ambulance? *If a large amount of fluid (i.e., greater than 500 cc) was given, it implies that patient's blood pressure was low and needed the fluid to support it. Alternatively, it could imply negligence on the ambulance crew's part.*
- Was the patient intubated (i.e., endotracheal intubation)?
- What were the indications for intubation? *Was there apnea? Was it to support the airway in the case of bleeding, emesis, or decreased level of consciousness?*
- Was the ambulance crew member who performed the intubation trained and certified in this procedure?
- Did the ambulance crew member examine the patient's lung and abdomen to ensure the correct placement of the endotracheal tube?
- Were any medications administered to the patient by people at the scene?
- Were any medications administered by the ambulance crew?
- Who in the ambulance crew made the decision to administer the medication?
- Who in the ambulance crew administered it?
- Was the ambulance crew instructed to administer medication by an MD at the hospital, or did they use their own judgment?
- Did the ambulance crew administer medication following a protocol? For example, did they give an opiate antagonist, a 50% Dextrose solution, Narcan, and insulin to a patient who is unconscious?
- Who provided that protocol?
- Was CPR ever used?
- Was the crew certified in BLS, CPR, or ALS (advanced life support)?
- Were there other victims at the scene?
- If there were other victims, what was their condition?
- If there were other victims, were they cared for (or transported) by the same ambulance crew?

Q **What should be asked about an automotive accident?**

- What was the condition of the car(s) involved in the accident?
- Did the patient's car have seat belts?

- Were seat belts used by the patient?
- Was the car equipped with air bags? Which seats had air bags associated with them? Were they driver's side, passenger side, or side curtain air bags?
- Were air bags deployed?
- Where was the patient seated in the car?
- Did the patient hit and fracture the windshield? *This is sometimes noted as a "spider-webbed" or, more colloquially, a "spidered" windshield.*
- Was the steering wheel broken by impact with the driver's body?
- Was the collision head-on with a stationary object?
- Was the collision head-on with another moving car?
- Was the collision a "side impact" or "T-Bone" impact?
- Where did the car(s) impact?
- Were there other victims in the car?
- How severe were their injuries?
- Were there any fatalities? *There is a close correlation between the injuries of victims in the same car. Severe injuries in one occupant of the car correlates with severe injuries in another occupant. A fatality in a car imposes a high risk of severe or fatal injury in another occupant.*
- Was the patient ejected from the car? *The mortality rate of patients ejected from a vehicle during an accident is extremely high.*
- Did the car roll over? *Rollovers are associated with a high rate of cervical spine injuries.*
- Did the patient make any statements about the cause of the accident at the scene? *Statements made immediately after the accident are unlikely to be calculated to shift liability or amplify injury. Therefore, they should be given greater credence than statements made later in the course of treatment or after consultation with family, friends, or legal counsel.*
- Did the ambulance crew make any mention of the smell of alcohol on the breath of the patient or driver? *This is sometimes noted as "+ ETOH" or "+ AOB."*
- Did the ambulance crew make any statements about the conditions of the road (e.g., wet, icy, or dry), the weather conditions (e.g., rainy, cold, overcast, foggy, sunny, and clear), or the lighting conditions (e.g., dark, light, bright sunshine, and glare)?

- Are any witnesses of the accident mentioned?
- Were there any "good samaritans" that provided aid or called the ambulance at the scene mentioned in the ACR? *These people are possible witnesses to the mechanics of the accident, or condition of the patient before or after the time of the accident.*

Q   **What should be asked about a "slip and fall" case?**

- Where exactly did the accident occur?
- Where was the patient when the ambulance arrived?
- How did the patient get from the scene of the accident to where the ambulance found him or her?
- Were any witnesses to the accident identified?
- What where the patient's complaints at the scene?
- Did the patient state the mechanism of the injury?
- Did the ambulance crew member record the mechanism of injury?
- Was the patient able to ambulate at the scene?
- Did the patient have to be carried on a gurney?
- What was the patient's mental status upon arrival of the ambulance?
- Was there a report that the patient had lost consciousness? *This is usually indicated "+ LOC."*
- Was the patient conscious at the time of arrival of the ambulance?
- Was the patient alert, obtunded, or somnolent?
- Was the patient able to recall what occurred at the time of the accident?
- Could the patient recall events just before the time of the accident? *Significant head injuries can result in "retrograde amnesia" (i.e., the inability to remember events that occurred before the accident).*

CHAPTER 11

Emergency Department Record

WHAT IS THE ED RECORD?

The *emergency department record* is the memorialization of the patient's interaction with the hospital's emergency medical department (or ED). The record begins when the patient crosses the threshold of the ED and ends upon discharge from the ED.

Who creates the ED record?

The ED record is a collaborative effort that may include information from the following individuals:

- **ED clerk**. The *ED clerk* collects demographic, insurance, and billing data.
- **Triage nurse**. Triage can be defined as the medical screening of patients to determine their relative priority for treatment. The *triage nurse* is a nurse employed by the ED who is assigned the task of triage of incoming patients. The triage nurse determines the patient's initial need for services, elicits the initial complaint, performs a cursory evaluation of the patient, and takes the first set of vital signs.
- **ED nurse**. The *ED nurse* is responsible for a more extensive interview and examination of the patient once the patient is in a treatment room in the ED. She may also perform an ECG, order X-rays, draw blood, or acquire a urine sample for

analysis. The ED nurse is also responsible for "picking up" (carrying out) physician orders and administering medications.

- **ED physician**. The *ED physician* obtains a history, performs a physical examination, evaluates clinical tests, makes a preliminary diagnosis, and determines the disposition of the patient (i.e., admission or discharge). The ED physician may begin therapy in the ED or perform emergency procedures such as suturing, setting fractures, and inserting chest tubes.
- **Consultant**. In the case of life-threatening emergencies, an expert *consultant* may be called to the ED to help render a diagnosis, suggest a therapy, or perform a procedure. The consultant will write a note and describe his or her examination, findings, and recommendations. This note is often written on a separate sheet of paper and appended to the ED note. If a medical or surgical procedure is performed, the consultant will describe the procedure, the results, and care plan. If the ED note suggests that a consultant was called, is there a corresponding consultant's note on the ED chart? If not, where is it?

While the majority of the important information will come from the nurses' and physician's notes, simple identification data, such as arrival and discharge time, age, home address, or insurance company can contradict patient statements or change liability.

Q

What is contained in the ED record?

A

The ED record includes the following components:

- Demographics (i.e., name, date of birth, address, next of kin, etc.)
- Billing information (i.e., responsible party, insured, dependent, name of insurance company, policy number, and employer)
- Time of arrival (i.e., when the patient registered with the clerk)
- Time of treatment (written by the treating nurse in the ED)
- Time of discharge
- Physician's orders
- Nurse's notes
- Medications (i.e., name, dose, route of administration and administration times, and name of nurse who administered the medication)
- Chief complaint

- History of present illness
- Focused physical examination
- Current medications
- Allergies
- Preliminary tests (e.g., laboratory, radiological, electrocardiographic)
- Preliminary diagnosis and plan
- Disposition (e.g., discharged, admitted, eloped from ED, or deceased)
- Discharge instructions (e.g., wound care, instructions on taking medications, instructions on when to follow up with physicians, what to do in case condition becomes worse, etc.)
- Post-discharge notes and follow-up notes (e.g., any calls from the ED to the patient regarding his or her condition, or results of X-rays or other tests performed in the ED but not available till after discharge). *Alternatively, the patient may have called the ED and reported some change in status or asked for advice on care for his or her injury or illness.*

Q **What should be asked about the ED record?**

- Who first saw the patient? *Usually a triage nurse will see the patient before the patient is officially checked into the ED.*
- Did the triage nurse record the patient's original complaint?
- Did the triage nurse use the patient's own words?
- Does the nurse state to whom she referred the patient (e.g., physician, NP, PA, or nurse in the ED)? *Did the physician or nurse indicate in the note some suspicion of veracity of the patient? Were words such as "patient reports," "patient alleges," or "patient claims" used in the chief complaint?*
- How did the patient arrive at the ED? Did he or she arrive by car or by ambulance or walk in?
- Did the ED clerk or nurse record who accompanied the patient to the ED (e.g., parent, spouse, or friend)? (Potential witnesses)
- When did the patient go to the ED in relation to the time of the medical event or accident?
- How long did the ambulance or private vehicle take to arrive at the ED?
- Was there any unusual delay in responding to the scene or during the transfer to the ED?

- Did the emergency service workers stop the ambulance to perform needed emergency treatments?
- Did the ambulance experience any traffic delays?
- Was the patient seen in the ED the same day of the accident or injury or was the visit delayed?
- When the patient arrived, was he or she able to ambulate unassisted?
- Was the patient given a splint or cast?
- Did the patient use an assistive device such as a cane, walker, or a wheelchair?
- Did the patient come in on a stretcher?
- Was the patient immobilized with a cervical collar or on a long board, or did he or she have another type of spinal immobilization? *A patient's disability upon arrival to the ED should give some insight into the severity of the illness/injury and subsequent disability.*
- Was the patient awake, alert, or even conscious on arrival at the ED?
- Did the patient report the complaints or did a friend or family member?
- Did the patient speak English?
- Did the patient need a translator?
- Did the patient bring his own translator, or did someone at the hospital translate?
- How fluent was the translator in English or the patient's language?
- Were there any delays in treatment? If the visit did not occur the same day as the accident, is there any reason reported for why the patient waited to go to the ED? For example, does the record say "the patient's symptoms became worse" or "patient instructed to go to ED by his attorney?"
- Were there any complaints by the plaintiff? Were these the same complaints that were documented by the EMTs or ambulance crew?
- Do the patient's complaints differ between the ED record, the in-patient record, or the record from the outpatient clinic or private physician's office?
- What injuries are recorded on first presentation?
- Were other injuries discovered after admission?

- Were the injuries definitively diagnosed, or were they just suspected in the ED?
- Was the diagnosis confirmed with objective tests such as an X-ray, CT scan, or peritoneal lavage and aspiration?
- Does the ED record mention if the patient was wearing his seat belt at the time of the accident?
- Was the patient described as having been restrained at the time of the accident?
- Did the car have air bags?
- Were the air bags deployed?
- If the air bag was deployed, was this fact mentioned in the ambulance call report? Is it mentioned later in subsequent records?
- Has there been any change in the story?
- Did the patient report a loss of consciousness at the accident scene?
- If the patient did report loss of consciousness, did it occur before or after the accident?
- Does the medical record reflect any history of unexplained syncope, cardiac arrhythmias, seizure disorder, or medications that could result in syncope or seizure disorder (e.g., hypoglycemic agents, insulin, blood pressure medications, sedatives, sleeping pills, and antihistamines)?
- What was the patient's level of consciousness in the ED? *In cases of negligence where an appropriate history is in question or there is disagreement over informed consent, assessing the level of consciousness in the ED is important. A patient described as A&OX3 (i.e., alert and oriented to person, place, and time) should know who he is, where he is, and the date. But this does not describe the higher functions of judgment. Check the physician and nurse's notes for descriptions of sleepiness, somnolence, lack of arousability, or any suggestions of intoxication, hypoglycemia, hypoxia, etc. The Glasgow Coma Scale is a way of reporting a level of consciousness. The scale ranges from 1 to 15. A score of 15 indicates a patient who is alert and answers questions appropriately. A score of three indicates a patient in a coma.*
- Did the patient have any pre-existing medical conditions? *Some medical conditions can either cause an accident or can*

cause disabilities that are later blamed on the accident. Look for a history of seizure disorder, strokes, and transient ischemic attacks (potential for raising questions of liability), diabetes and hypoglycemia, and visual impairment such as myopia, glaucoma, cataracts, retinitis, or macular degeneration. Hearing impairment or history of vertigo may suggest an alternate theory of liability.

- Was the patient taking any medications on admission? *A review of the patient's medication on admission to the ED may give clues to medical conditions that may have caused an accident. Additionally, some medications may suggest that the patient was suffering from a condition prior to the accident. This condition may later be claimed to have been caused by the accident. Look for anxiolytics, sedatives, tranquilizers, antidepressants, and narcotics that may cause drowsiness. Many drugs have significant side effects that could impair a patient. If the reviewer is unfamiliar with the medications listed in the medical chart, he or she should consult a pharmacology text or the Physician's Desk Reference. The use of narcotics or other pain relievers raises questions about pre-existing chronic pain conditions. Eye drops use raises issues concerning visual acuity. A history of being on antidepressants may be significant if the patient claims to have become depressed as a result of the accident (as a new condition instead of acknowledging the existence of a pre-existing condition).*

- **Impairment:** *ED charts may record suspicion of impairment by drugs or alcohol. Statements such as " + ETOH," "INTOX," or "AOB" (alcohol on breath) may be especially significant in cases of accidents involving the operation of motor vehicles and machinery, or a "trip and fall." Look for a report of blood alcohol level or urinalysis. Be careful to check the time of the testing for alcohol and drugs. Testing for a blood alcohol level many hours after admission may give a misleadingly low level. Similarly, a urine toxicology screen taken after narcotics are administered in the ED may lead the reviewer to erroneously suspect drug intoxication as a cause of the accident. Other causes of impairment include head injuries, dementia, hypoxia, low blood pressure, low blood sugar, cardiac arrhythmias, and mental illness. Check previous diagnoses, the ECG, the arterial blood gas, blood pressure, and so on. The level of mental impair-*

*ment has significance when there are issues of liability for acci-
dents, appropriateness of informed consent, or when a patient is
given instructions on discharge to follow up and fails to.*

Q **Did the patient describe the mechanism of injury?**

- Is the mechanism described the same way in the ambulance
  call report, ED notes, and hospital notes?
- Did the patient change his story as time progressed, when the
  possibility of benefiting from a lawsuit became apparent?
- Does the mechanism seem to agree with the resulting
  injury?
- What symptoms did the patient experience while in the ED?
- Did the patient's behavior agree with the extent and severity
  of reported injuries, or did the ED personnel document
  behaviors that would cast doubt on the severity of the
  injuries?

Q **What types of laboratory and X-ray testing were done
in the ED?**

- Were the appropriate X-rays taken based on the plaintiff's
  complaints?
- Were X-rays read by the radiologist or only by the ED physician initially?
- Does the X-ray interpretation by the ED physician and the
  radiologist agree? *Make sure that the final radiological report
  agrees with the interpretation by the ED physician. A radiologist must review all ED X-rays. Sometimes the final radiological
  report is not added to the ED chart until several days after the
  patient has been discharged.*
- If there was a missed diagnosis, did the ED physician call
  the patient and ask him to return to the ED or another
  physician's office for evaluation or treatment? *While the
  results of most laboratory tests such as complete blood count
  and urinalysis are available within a few hours, some test
  results may take a few days to be reported. It is important to
  determine when these tests were completed, when the results
  were available, and what the ED physician did about abnormal
  or dangerous test results.*

Q
A

Did the patient report any headaches in the ED?

The majority of headaches are caused by muscular spasms. ED physicians, however, are obligated to "rule out" the rare but potentially fatal causes of headache, such as intracerebral bleeding, venous thrombosis, or meningitis.

- Did the physician ask for a complete history of the headache? *Sudden intense headaches are very suspicious and should prompt further testing.*
- Did the physician elicit a full neurologic history by asking about weakness, numbness, difficulty speaking, or visual disturbance?
- Did the physician examine the retina looking for papilledema? *Papilledema is a sign of increased intracerebral pressure.*
- Was a complete neurologic exam performed?
- Was a CT, MRI, or lumbar puncture performed?
- Was there any mention of the patient seeming to be dull, slow, sleepy, or obtunded?
- Did the patient complain of nausea, vomiting, dizziness, or visual disturbance? *These are symptoms of increased intracranial pressure.*
- Did these symptoms prompt immediate evaluation with a CT?
- Was a neurologist or neurosurgeon called to evaluate the patient urgently?

Did the patient report any chest pain in the ED?

The dangerous causes of chest pain include heart attack, aortic aneurysm, and pulmonary embolism. The ED physician must distinguish these causes from the indigestion and chest wall inflammation that make up the majority of the causes of chest pain.

- Did the triage nurse or ED physician bring the patient into the ED immediately after the patient reported chest pain, or did he or she wait in the waiting area?
- Was an ECG performed on the patient? *There must be a very good reason for an ECG not to be done on a person complaining of chest pain. The ECG is a quick and easy test to perform. It does not have any risks associated with it and provides important information.*

- Was a full history of the pain evaluated?
- Was the pain associated with other suspicious symptoms such as shortness of breath, dizziness, nausea, or vomiting?
- Was a chest X-ray ordered?
- Were serum blood tests performed for cardiac enzymes?
- Was an echocardiogram performed?
- Was a cardiologist consulted? When?
- Were the cardiologist's orders followed?
- Was the patient given an aspirin?
- Was the patient started on a blood thinner such as unfractionated heparin or low molecular weight heparin?

Q **What kind of wound care did the patient receive in the ED?**

- What type of wound was it (e.g., laceration, crush injury, burn, avulsion)?
- Was a full examination of the extremities' sensation and motor function obtained before anesthesia and wound closure?
- If the wound was in the chest or abdomen, were X-rays taken to rule out puncture of the peritoneum or hemithorax?
- Was it appropriate for this wound to be closed in the ED?
- Should the wound have been evaluated or explored under anesthesia in the operating room?
- Was it an ED physician who closed the wound?
- Was it a surgeon or a plastic surgeon who closed the wound?
- Was the physician handling the wound appropriately trained in this area?
- Should a consultation have been called?
- Was the wound appropriately irrigated?
- What was used to irrigate the wound (e.g., water, normal saline, or hydrogen peroxide)?
- How much irrigant was used?
- Was the wound carefully explored for foreign bodies?
- Was an X-ray taken to look for foreign bodies or broken bones under the wound?
- Was the wound tetanus prone? *In other words, did the wound have a lot of devitalized tissue or foreign body contamination?*
- Was the patient queried about his or her last tetanus vaccination?
- Did the patient receive an injection of tetanus antibody or a tetanus toxoid?
- Did the patient receive antibiotics?

- Were appropriate follow-up instructions given to care for the wound and was a follow-up appointment with a physician scheduled?

Q   **Did the patient report any abdominal pain in the ED?**

- Was a complete history taken of the pain?
- Did the ED physician elicit a history of dietary habits, weight loss, or weight gain and changes in bowel movements?
- Was a menstrual history taken?
- Was a pregnancy test performed on any women of child-bearing age?
- Was a medication history taken? *For example, was there any history of gastrointestinal bleeding with nonsteroidal anti-inflammatory drugs, constipation with antidepressants and opiates, etc.*
- Was a complete physical exam performed? *This exam should include a stool guaiac for occult blood, auscultation of the abdomen for bruits, and evaluation of the iliac/femoral pulses to rule out an aortic aneurysm.*
- Were X-rays of the chest and abdomen taken?
- Were a complete blood count, hematocrit test, and hemoglobin test performed?
- Was an abdominal sonogram available?
- Was an abdominal sonogram performed?
- Who read the sonogram?
- If a sonogram was performed, was it read by the technologist, ED physician, or radiologist? *Sonograms are quickly performed, risk-free tests that can yield a great amount of information.*
- Was a diagnosis of appendicitis appropriately evaluated? *In the elderly, especially those with a history of vascular disease or heart failure, the diagnosis of mesenteric ischemia should be entertained.*
- Was a surgeon called to evaluate the patient?
- Was the patient discharged with appropriate instructions on what to do if the pain persisted?
- What was the patient told to do if the pain got worse?
- Did the ED physician inquire if the patient was able to return without trouble? *A patient who does not have the network (friends and family members) or resources (telephone, car, and*

*access to public transportation) to easily return to the ED
should not be discharged, but should be observed carefully until
a diagnosis is made.*

Q **Did the patient come to the ED with pneumonia or another
severe infection?**

- When was the diagnosis made?
- Was a chest X-ray taken?
- If a chest X-ray was taken, who read the chest X-ray?
- Was a CT scan performed?
- If a CT scan was performed, who read the CT scan?
- Was a white blood cell count performed?
- Was culture and sensitivity performed on the appropriate tissue or fluid (e.g., blood, spinal fluid, urine, and wound)?
- Was a gram stain performed on the sputum to help guide antibiotic therapy?
- Was an orthostatic blood pressure test performed?
- Was pulse oximetry performed?
- Was an arterial blood gas test performed?
- What antibiotics were prescribed?
- If antibiotics were prescribed, when were they prescribed?
- Were antibiotic allergies inquired about?
- If antibiotic allergies were inquired about, was this recorded in the chart?
- If antibiotics were prescribed, were they appropriate for the infection?
- If antibiotics were prescribed, when were they administered?
- Was there a significant delay in administration of antibiotics (i.e., within less than two hours from diagnosis)?
- Did a delay in administering the antibiotics result in harm to the patient?

Q **Did the patient experience cardiac or respiratory arrest in
the ED?**

- When did the arrest occur?
- What was the patient's condition before the arrest?
- Was the arrest foreseeable?
- Where did the arrest occur (i.e., in the waiting room, triage station, or ED)?

- Was the arrest witnessed?
- Who witnessed the arrest (e.g., a family member, nurse, resident, and/or attending physician)?
- Who started the resuscitation?
- Was an attending physician present during the resuscitation?
- Was a resuscitation protocol followed?
- Were appropriate medications and procedures used?
- Were there any difficulties during the resuscitation (e.g., equipment failure, lack of appropriate medications, complication to procedures, inability to intubate the patient)?

Q   **Were there any consultant notes in the ED?**

- Was a consultant called from the ED?
- When was the call made?
- Who was called?
- When did he or she respond?
- What did the consultant find after the examination?
- Does that diagnosis agree with the ED physician's diagnosis?
- What recommendations did the consultant make?
- Did the ED physician put those recommendations on the order sheet?
- If there were consultant's recommendations on the order sheet, were they acted on by the nursing staff?
- How long did it take the nurses to "pick up" the order?
- If there were delays in execution of an order, were they appropriate?
- What was the patient's condition after the consultant's procedure (if any?)

Q   **Did the patient receive discharge instructions?**

- Were they written or oral?
- Are there copies of the written instructions in the chart?
- Did the patient sign the instruction sheet acknowledging that he or she understood the instructions?
- Did the chart indicate the patient's condition, level of alertness, or ability to comprehend when the instructions were given?
- Did the instructions properly indicate how to care for the medical condition?

- Did the discharge instructions include what prescriptions were given?
- Did the discharge instructions include what the doses and intervals of administration were for the prescriptions?
- Did the ED physician give the patient names of physicians to follow up with?
- Did the ED physician consult with the follow-up physician?
- Did the ED physician make an appointment for the patient?
- Was the patient given a physician's name and contact information?
- Was the patient instructed to seek care from his Primary Medical Doctor?

Q **Did the patient call the ED for any reason before or after the ED admission?**

- Did the patient seek advice from the ED physician or nurses?
- Were any suggestions made for follow-up care?
- Did the patient complain of any medication side effects or complications of the ED treatment?
- When did the patient call?
- Did the patient call more than once?
- What did the nurse or physician tell the patient?
- Was a return to the ED suggested?
- Did the ED physician or nurse attempt to call the patient about a possible problem regarding lab tests, X-rays, or biopsy results?
- How many times did the ED staff try to contact the patient?
- Were letters or telegrams sent requesting the patient to follow up?

CHAPTER 12

Admission Note

Q What is an admission note?

A The *admission note* is usually the first note after the emergency department (ED) record. It contains a comprehensive summary of the patient's reason for admission, current condition, medical history, and plan of treatment. (See Figure 12.1.)

Q Who is the author of the admission note?

A The admission note can be written by an intern, resident, or attending physician.

Q What information does the admission note contain?

A The data in the admission note should be pertinent and relevant. The admission note should include sufficient information necessary to provide the care and services required to address the patient's conditions and needs. As such, the specific data could be different for pediatrics, obstetrics, coronary care, psychiatry, and other patient populations. Specifically, the note should contain the following subheadings:

    i.   Chief Complaint
   ii.   History of Present Illness
  iii.   Past Medical History

Doe, JANE
DOB : 6/14/32

Physician Notes

Date/ Time	
	ATTENDING ADMISSION NOTE
	CC:
12/8/03	The pt is a 75 y/o W ♀ c̄ PMH of COPD who c/o difficulty swallowing solids for 3 weeks AND a 40 lb weight loss over the past 4 months.
	HPI: The patient was in her USOH until 3 weeks ago when she noticed it was difficult to swallow solid food. The difficulty increased AND she noticed that food seemed to get stuck in her throat. She denies ___ Difficulty sleeping, fever, chest surgery, hoarseness of voice, visual ___ neck injuries or masses. The patient reports that her clothes are very lose on her, and when she weighed herself she noticed she had lost 40 lbs. She denies dieting.
	PMH - Diagnosed c̄ COPD 5 years ago. ⊖ surgeries, 3 children, NVD
	Social hx : 2 PPD smoking x 40 years 3-4 mixed drinks / week Lives Alone. Never married.
	Occupational hx: worked as a secretary in an insurance company x 40 years
	Family hx: history of stomach CA in mother Father c̄ CAD No siblings children A+W
	P.E. VS P: 94 R: 12 BP 110/80 T: 99°
	HEENT - WNL Neck - supple ⊕ shotty nodes in ant. cerical chains ⊖ masses, ⊖ thyromegaly chest - clear -Bilaterally.

Figure 12.1   An Example of an Admission Note

Chief Complaint.   The *chief complaint* (sometimes abbreviated CC) is a brief statement of the medical issues that brought the patient to the attention of his physician or the ED. Physicians are encouraged during their training to use the patient's own words when writing the chief complaint. The following are some examples of chief complaints:

- I've been short of breath for three days.
- I've been having chest pain for the past hour.
- I've had pain and swelling of my knee for a week.

History of Present Illness.   *The history of present illness* (sometimes abbreviated as HPI) is a deeper explanation of the chief complaint. The physician explores the complaint by asking probing, open-ended questions, allowing the patient to tell his or her story. The HPI should explain when the condition seemed to start, how long it lasted, how much it affected the patient, how severe the complaint was, and what was done about it. The following are some typical questions asked in the HPI:

- When did the pain begin?
- How long have you had this numbness?
- Can you describe the sensation you have in your chest?
- When did you last speak to your physician?
- Did the medication you took make the pain better or worse?
- Was the chest pain associated with any other symptoms such as shortness of breath or dizziness?

Past Medical History.   The *past medical history* is a data set that seeks to record all prior medical, surgical, or psychiatric complaints. The physician is encouraged to record, as specifically as possible, all interactions with the health care system such as places and dates of prior hospitalizations, surgeries, X-rays, biopsies, lab tests, and therapies and the responses to those therapies. The past medical history adds data to the history of current illness, helps the physician make sense of the patient's current complaints, and helps the physician to create an accurate diagnosis.

Family History.   The *family history* examines the medical histories of first- and second-degree relatives as well as people that the patient lives with. In some cases, diseases with a genetic component can be discovered. In others, risk factors for certain diseases such as heart disease or breast cancer can help the physician determine the patient's risk for those diseases or plan diagnostic tests to rule them out. When asking about those persons the patient lives with, but is not related to by blood, such as a spouse or significant other, the physician may be looking for evidence of contagious diseases or common exposures to toxins or tainted food.

Social History.   The content of a patient's *social history* varies from institution to institution, but it should contain the following histories:

- History of use of legal and illegal drugs, alcohol, and tobacco use.
- Sexual history. *Evidence of sexual dysfunction may be an indicator of other diseases such as diabetes, pituitary disease, or depression. The sexual history also seeks to find high-risk sexual behaviors that may lead to sexually transmitted diseases. The physician also explores the home life of the patient for physical abuse or neglect from a partner.*
- Employment history, especially looking for occupational exposures to toxins or microorganisms. *Some examples of this are ship builders and asbestosis, and farming and zoonostic diseases or exposure to pesticides.*
- Travel history. *Has the patient traveled to countries or areas where there are endemic diseases such as malaria, dysentery, or viral encephalitides? Has the patient been on jet planes for many hours, putting him at risk for deep venous thrombosis or pulmonary embolism?*

Review of Systems.   The *review of systems* (sometimes abbreviated as ROS) is a systematic screening of the eight major organ systems of the human body. The purpose of this review is to prompt the patient (and the physician) to examine seemingly nonrelated complaints such as weight loss and constipation, which could possibly indicate a bowel carcinoma, or skin lesion and neurologic deficit, which could possibly indicate a melanoma with brain metastasis. The ROS should be a component of every comprehensive history and physical examination.

The following are organ systems that are typically reviewed in the review of systems:

- Neurological
- Psychological
- Endocrine
- Gastrointestinal
- Respiratory
- Cardiovascular
- Rheumatological
- Integument (skin, hair, and nails)

Current Medications.   A list of all the current medications the patient takes is essential. This list should include dosages and intervals as well as the indications for the medication. The *current medications* list should include all medications taken by the patient including prescription medications, over-the-counter medications, vitamins, herbal remedies, cathartics, enemas, poultices, or other nontraditional therapies. These non-physician-prescribed medications may contribute to illness, interfere with more effective therapies, or point to an illness or complaint that the patient had failed to mention because of a memory lapse or embarrassment.

Allergies.   The *allergies* section of an admission note lists all allergies that the patient is aware of. The physician should not only question about allergies to medications but also to foods, chemicals, or other organic or inorganic substances. The physician should record not only the fact of an allergy but also the characteristics of the allergic reaction. For example, an allergic history may include comments like "patient reports diffuse rash over body 12 hours after taking ampicillin by mouth" or "patient states she became short of breath and unconscious after eating shellfish."

The Physical Examination.   In the ED and progress note, physicians can legitimately perform a "focused physical exam." The admission note should record a comprehensive physical examination that includes the following information:

- Vital Signs (including orthostatic blood pressures when indicated)
- Head
- Eyes and Fundi

- Ears, Nose, and Throat
- Neck
- Chest
- Breasts (on male patients also)
- Heart
- Abdomen
- Genitals
- Pelvic Exam
- Digital Rectal Exam (with test for occult blood in stool)
- Extremities
- Mental Status exam
- Neurological
- Vascular
- Skin and Integument

Laboratory Testing.   While little medical evidence exists to justify a standard battery of "admission tests," some testing is routinely done on admission. Typically, this laboratory work includes the following tests:

- Electrocardiogram (ECG)
- Serum Electrolytes (sodium, potassium, chloride, etc.)
- Complete Blood Count (CBC)
- Chest X-ray
- Any number of other tests may be ordered on admission depending on the diagnosis. These tests may include lab work as diverse as viral titers, blood cultures, CTs of the head, or prostate ultrasounds.

Analysis.   The *analysis* is the part of the admission note where the physician evaluates the history as well as findings from the physical exam and laboratory tests. The result of this analysis should be a diagnosis or, at least, a group of possible diagnoses (also called a differential diagnosis).

Plan.   The *plan* is a road map, prepared by the physician, for either further diagnostic procedures or therapeutic interventions. Further diagnostic tests are aimed at confirming a suspected diagnosis. The diagnostic tests may include a consultation with one or more specialists. The therapeutic plan should contain specific treatment strategies (e.g., "IV Penicillin G for 10 days" or "transfer to surgery for immediate cholecystectomy").

Q **What should be asked about the admission note?**

- Who wrote the admission note?
- Was it an intern, resident, or attending physician who wrote the admission note? *In academic institutions, the admission history and physical examination may be written by a medical student, physician's assistant, or nurse practitioner. These notes need to be countersigned by an attending physician who examined the patient and verified the veracity of the notes contents.*
- Is the note complete?
- What is missing from the history or physical exam?
- Was any part of the physical exam deferred for any reason? *Examinations that are commonly deferred are rectal, breast, and gynecological exams. These exams may be either the patient's or the physician's choice.*
- If any part of the physical exam was deferred, why was it deferred?
- If there was a deferral, was it appropriate?
- If there was a deferral, was the patient harmed by the lack of full examination?
- Have all the various subheadings of a complete exam been included?
- Are any positive findings mentioned in the history, physical examination, or laboratory results not addressed in the assessment and plan? *It is not uncommon for a patient to enter the hospital with more than one significant medical problem. Often, the most obvious (or most critical) problem is addressed and the other problems overlooked or ignored. Ignoring signs of occult cancer, heart disease, or infection is not uncommon.*
- Do all tests and treatments mentioned in the treatment plan section of the admission note appear in the physician's orders?
- Are any of the drugs ordered in the treatment plan also included on the list of drugs the patient is allergic to?
- Are any of the drugs ordered in the treatment plan contraindicated for this patient? *Many drugs cannot be safely administered to some patients (e.g., Viagra and patients with heart disease, Thalidomide and pregnant patients, Tetracycline and infant patients, and Gentamicin and patients with renal*

failure). An easy way to find this out is to cross-reference the medications with their contraindications listed in the Physician's Desk Reference.

- Was the old chart available on this patient?
- Did the admitting physician seek out and review an old chart?
- Had the patient been treated by a physician before?
- Did the admitting physician attempt to ask the patient's private physician about prior diagnoses or therapies?
- Was an interpreter used?
- Who interpreted for the patient? *Did a family member or close friend interpret? Using a family member or close friend as an interpreter can present problems for the physician as the patient may not want to be completely forthright about certain aspects of his behavior when he knows a family member or friend will hear about it. Physicians should seek out and use a disinterested interpreter when performing an in-depth history. Errors or omissions in the patient's history may be attributed to this mistake.*

CHAPTER **13**

Physician Order Sheet

Q **What is the physician order sheet?**

A The *physician order sheet* is the main mode of communication between the physician caring for the patient and the nursing and clerical staff. It is a written record of all orders and requests made by the physician about the care of a patient. (See Figure 13.1).

Q **Who writes physician orders?**

A Physician orders are written by the physician caring for the patient. Having more than one professional writing physician orders on the patient is seen as a dangerous practice. Hospitals insist that only the treating physician write the orders to avoid redundancy and confusion. Nurses and other physicians are usually prohibited from writing on this sheet. If a consultant believes the patient would benefit from a particular medication or therapy, he or she is obliged to write suggestions in the consultation report or speak with the treating physician directly. Similarly, if the primary nurse feels the patient may benefit from a particular diagnostic or therapeutic intervention, he or she is obliged to call the physician and request an order.

Verbal Orders. In the situation where the physician is not physically able to write the order, he or she may give a "telephone" order, or "verbal order." For a verbal order, the nurse

	Acme Hospital Physician Orders	Patient Name: Doe, John DOB: 12/15/55 Medical Record No.: 162306 Nursing Station: 3A	
Date/ Time			**Nurses Initials**
3/17/04 13:00 hrs	1) ADMIT to MEDICINE 2) DIAGNOSIS: EXASCERBATION OF ASTHMA R/o PNEUMONIA		

	3) DIET: 2gm Na+ diet, 2000 CAL
	4) VITAL SIGNS @ 4 hrs
	5) PEAK flow Q 4 hrs
	6) LABS:
	          CBC
	          SMA-12
	          Sputum for Gram STAIN + C+S
	          ABG ON ROOM AIR
	          BLOOD C+S X 2
	7) RADIOLOGY - CXRAY UPRIGHT + LATERAL
	8) MEDS:
	          O₂ 35% VIA VENTI MASK
	          Azithromycin 500mg PO STAT
	          PROVENTIL MDI TT PUFFS Q 4 hrs
	          PREDNISONE 40mg PO BID		

	9) ConsulT Pulmonology iN AM.		
	J. Smith, MD) BEEPER #312		
	Please Press Firmly Use Pen Only		

Figure 13.1   Example of a Physician Order Sheet

transcribes the physician's request onto the order sheet noting the time and circumstances of the verbal order. The physician is usually responsible for countersigning the verbal order within a time period specified by hospital policy.

What does the physician order sheet contain?

A physician order sheet usually has three columns. The first column is labeled Time/ Date. The second column is the widest and is labeled Order, and the third column is labeled Signature. In the first column, the physician records the time and date of the order. In the second column, the physician writes exactly what he wants accomplished, and the third column is for the nurse to record the time and date the order was carried out and her signature. The physician's orders should encompass every aspect of the patient's care, from the setting of care (e.g., "Admit to Intensive care unit") to the diet (e.g., "2 gm sodium diet") to restrictions on activity (e.g., "strict bed rest").

Q

A

How are they organized?

Physician orders follow a standard format. On admission, the physician writes orders that describe the care and setting for the patient, as well as the patient's diet, medications, and diagnostic tests. Further, the orders may request specialist consultations. Every order must be explicit as to how, how much, when, and where. For example, an order for a medication must include the following information:

- Time and date of the order
- Name of the medication
- Dosage of the medication
- Interval of administration
- Route of administration

Q

A

Who is supposed to respond to physician orders?

The hospital ward clerk and the nurses respond to the physician's orders. The ward clerk is responsible for requesting consultations and diagnostic tests. The nurse usually handles all other tasks. As the orders are "picked up," the nurse or ward clerk checks off the order and signs his or her name.

Q

What should be asked about the physician order sheet?

- Who wrote the orders? *What was the physician's name? What were his qualifications? Was it an intern, a resident, an attending physician, or a consulting physician?*
- Has more than one person been writing the physician orders? *If more than one person wrote them, was there a reason? Was there an emergent situation? Was there a mistake? Do orders contradict or contravene each other? Are any orders redundant?*

- When were the physician orders written? *Are they timed and dated appropriately? Was the order given in response to a patient care need? Was the order written in time to address that need?*
- Are the times and dates of the physician orders chronological? *Are there any gaps in the chronology? Is there irregularity in the chronology or are there gaps in the chronology that should prompt further investigation? Were orders written after the fact? Were orders written later to decrease or shift liability?*
- When did the nurse or ward clerk pick up the orders? *Were the physician orders legible? Were they accurate? Were they contradictory? If they were illegible, inaccurate, or contradictory, what did the nurse or ward clerk do? Is there a hospital policy on this situation? Were the orders clarified? Were the orders picked up in a reasonable amount of time? Was there a delay? Was the patient harmed by the delay? Were medication orders transcribed appropriately into the medication administration record (MAR)?*
- Did the nurses or ward clerk carry out the orders? *(In other words, was the medication given immediately after the order was picked up? To investigate this, compare the MAR with the physician order sheet. Was the consultant notified immediately after the order for a consultation was picked up? If there was a delay in carrying out the order, how long was the delay? Was the patient harmed by the delay? Who picked up the order? What were the qualifications of the nurse that picked up the order (e.g., LPN, RN, NP, etc.)? Was she qualified to carry out the order? Was she appropriately trained and certified to carry out the order? Were the nursing supervisors or managers aware of any inadequacy of training or experience in a nurse for a specific assignment? For example, did they send a labor and delivery nurse to work in the ED or ICU? Were the patient's responses to all medication and procedures recorded? If not, why?*
- Were the orders specific in their requests? *For example, did the orders specify name, dosage, interval, and route? Nonspecific orders make it difficult or impossible for the nurse to carry them out. Do the nurse's notes reflect a request for clarification? Were the ambiguous orders ignored? Could the name of the ordering physician be identified?*

- Were telephone orders recorded in the order sheet? *Is the physician who gave the orders identified? Is the date and time the order was given recorded? Was the order taken by the treating nurse or the ward clerk? Did the physician countersign the order? Is there any indication in the chart that the physician didn't give the order? Is there any indication in the chart that the nurse or ward clerk misunderstood the order?*

CHAPTER 14

Progress Note

Q   **What is a progress note?**

A   A *progress note* is the contemporaneous recording of clinically relevant events that occur between a patient and the health care system. This record is created by the physician caring for a patient in the inpatient setting. Progress notes are typically written on a daily basis after the physician examines the patient and reviews lab test results and X-ray reports. (See example in Figure 14.1).

Q   **Who writes the progress notes?**

A   Progress notes can appear in the medical chart under several headings such as attending progress note (APN), resident progress note (RPN), and intern progress note (IPN).

In the surgical arena, the progress notes may be called postoperative notes, post OP notes, or simply PON. The surgical progress note's title may also contain the amount of days since the surgery occurred. For example, a progress note three days after surgery would be labeled Post OP Day 3. Most patients will have only a single daily progress note. However, complex patients with many caregivers or in academic medical centers may have many daily progress notes. Each progress note will address the patient's condition, as seen through the eyes of the various medical and surgical specialists.

NAME: Doe, John
DOB: 10/4/51

Date/ Time	Physicians Notes	
12/7/03 10:00 AM	R PN	

S: Pt c/o ↑ SOB, ⊕ orthopnea, ⊖ CP
⊖ Dizziness ⊖ Nasea, ⊖ vomiting

O: HEENT – WNL
Neck ⊕ JVD, ⊖ masses
Chest – Lungs with rales ½ way up
lung fields Bilateral Ath,
– Heart – S₁ S₂ ⊕ S₃ (⊖MRG
– Breast – ⊖ masses on discharge
ABD – Soft, nontender, ⊕ BS
⊖ organomegaly

EXT – ⊖ clubbing ⊖ cyanosis
⊕ Edema / in Both Ankles
w? to mid calf

CXRAY – c/w pulmonary EDEMA
EKG – No interval change, LVH
CBC   H/ 12   10,000 WBC
/H 36   350,000 PLTS

A: Congestive heart failure

P: Lasix 40 mg IVP
Nitropaste, 1" to chest wall
Δ Diet to 2gm Na⁺
Consult Cardiology

A. Smith, MD
Beeper # 314

Figure 14.1   Example of a Progress Note

Q   What is contained in the progress note?

A   Progress notes may be long or short, complex or simple. Either
way, the progress note is written in the S.O.A.P. Note format. The
S.O.A.P. Note format has been the format of choice in American

medical schools for the last 30 years. S.O.A.P. stands for Subjective, Objective, Assessment, and Plan.

Subjective

Subjective findings are those "subjective issues" that the patient complains of. These issues typically include pain, shortness of breath, constipation, insomnia, or difficulty with ambulation. When recording subjective issues, the physician is encouraged to use the patient's own words and to be as complete as possible.

Objective

Objective findings include the patient's vital signs, inputs and outputs, results of the physical examination, lab tests, radiology reports, pathology reports, etc.

Assessment

The *assessment* is a record of the physician's thought processes in evaluating the import of test results. Do they point to a diagnosis? Do they indicate improvement or worsening of the patient's condition? Should alternated diagnoses be entertained?

Plan

The *plan* describes the treating physician's plans for further diagnostic tests, therapies, or specialty consultations. The typical format of the plan section is to single out each clinical complaint or diagnosis, and address it individually.

Q **What should be asked about the progress note?**

- Is the note legible? *If the note is not legible, the plaintiff can request a typed interpretation of the note from the defendant.*
- Is the note signed?
- Who wrote the note?
- Do all the progress notes written on the same day record the same information?
- Are important findings missed?
- Are important tests or events recorded in one note but not in another? *This would indicate a lack of communication between physicians or care teams.*
- Do incidents or events appear in the nursing notes that don't appear in the physician's notes?

- Did diagnostic or therapeutic plans in the progress note get entered in the physician's order form?
- Does the medical record show clear justification for diagnostic and therapeutic procedures?
- Do the progress notes contain negative comments about the actions of other physicians or nurses. Do they contain notes such as "I disagree with the infectious disease recommendation for triple antibiotics" or "I have called the orthopedic surgeon three times about this issue and he has not responded"?
- Do all the complaints in the subjective portion of the progress note get addressed in the plan portion of the progress note?
- Do all the significant findings in the objective portion of the note get addressed in the plan portion of the note?
- Are suggestions by consultants acknowledged in the assessment portion and followed in the plan portion of the progress note?
- If specialty consultants' suggestions are not followed, are appropriate reasons given?
- Are emergency findings noted and addressed?
- Does the note reflect calls to specialists in emergency situations?
- Does the clinical assessment support the decision for a referral?
- Is the referral requested in a timely manner according to the severity of the patient's condition?
- Do they record the name of a specialist?
- Does the note reflect the number of times a specialist was called and when?
- Were alternative providers called when the first provider didn't respond or responded negatively?
- Are the results of all lab and other diagnostics documented in the medical record? *Lack of documentation may indicate that the lab reports were not reviewed.*
- Does the progress note demonstrate that the practitioner reviewed the laboratory and diagnostic reports?
- Did the practitioner make appropriate treatment decisions based on the report findings?
- Were the lab reports reviewed within an appropriate period of time?

- Are the lab reports initialed and dated by the practitioner? *Does the physician have another system to ensure his review?*
- Are lab report "panic values" rapidly assessed and treated?
- Is information regarding current medications readily apparent from review of the record?
- Are changes to medication regimen noted as they occur?
- When medications appear to remain unchanged, does the record include documentation of, at least, annual review of the medications by the practitioner?
- When the patient is being seen by multiple practitioners, is there documentation of consideration of medication interaction?
- Is patient education addressed in the notes? *Education may correspond directly to the reason for the visit, to specific diagnosis-related issues, such as dietary instruction to reduce cholesterol, or be related to general health maintenance/ self-care/preventive health care, such as teaching monthly self breast examination, or other age- and gender-appropriate preventive recommendations.*
- Are examples of patient noncompliance documented?
- What has the physician done about the issue of noncompliance once it has been noted?
- Are preventive medical issues addressed in the chart? *The physician has an obligation to document preventive medical services. Each patient record should include documentation that preventive services were ordered and performed, or that the practitioner discussed preventive services with the patient and the patient chose to defer or refuse them. Practitioners may document that a patient sought preventive services from another practitioner (e.g., OB/GYN or private radiologist).*
- Are immunizations recorded? *The patient record should include documentation of immunizations administered from birth to present for patients 18 years and under. When prior records are unavailable, practitioners may document that a child's parent or guardian affirmed that immunizations were administered by another practitioner and the approximate age or date the immunizations were given.*
- Are consultation reports reviewed by the physician? *How is this documented?*

- If the consultation reports are not received after a referral to a specialist, does the primary care physician attempt to obtain those reports?
- Do subsequent visit notes reflect results of the consultation as may be pertinent to ongoing patient care?
- Do the specialist records include a consultation report/summary addressed to the referral source?
- Are any portions of the physical examination missing or deferred? The most commonly deferred examinations are: rectal, prostate, breast, and gynecological exams.
- Does the physician explain why these examinations are not completed?
- Is there documentation of a physician-patient discussion of risk associated with failure to fully examine the patient?
- Are the examinations referred to another physician (e.g., surgeon, gynecologist, oncologist, or urologist)?
- Is there documentation that the other physician performed these examinations (e.g., in pre-admission note or consultant's note)?

CHAPTER 15

Consultation Note

Q

What is a consultation note?

A

In the course of caring for a patient, a physician will often refer that patient to a consultant. This referral occurs because the original physician is unclear about a diagnosis or treatment plan and seeks the consultant's expert counsel, or when the patient requires a therapy or procedure that the original physician is unable to provide (e.g., radiation therapy or neurosurgery). The consultant is required to create a note documenting his findings and making recommendations for further diagnosis or treatment. This note is then sent to the physician who requested the consultation. In the outpatient setting, this note takes the form of a letter that is added to the originating physician's office notes. In the inpatient setting, the note is often handwritten on a consultation form that is added to the hospital chart.

Q

Who is the author of the consultation note?

A

The consultant writes the consultation note. The *consultant* is an experienced physician with specialized training in a medical subspecialty. In academic settings, an intern, resident, or fellow under supervision of the specialist or attending physician often writes the consultation note.

Q   **What should the consultation note contain?**

A   A consultation note should contain the following:

- Name of the service consulted (e.g., cardiology, orthopedics, infectious disease, etc.)
- Name of physician seeking consultation
- Reason for consultation
- Date of request
- Date of consultation
- History of illness in question
- Physical examination
- Description of any special procedures performed (e.g., endoscopy, visual field testing, or CT scan)
- Assessment or diagnosis
- Therapeutic or diagnostic plan
- Intention to follow up
- Consultant's signature

Q   **What should be asked about a consultation note?**

- When was the consultant requested? *Confirm this in physician order form.*
- When did the consultant respond to the request?
- Was there an unusual delay in the consultation? *In other words, was the delay greater than 24 hours in the inpatient setting or greater than 10 days in the outpatient setting?*
- Who was responsible for the delay? *Patient? Requesting physician? Consultant?*
- Did the patient's condition deteriorate due to the delay?
- What are the qualifications of the consultant?
- Is the consultant qualified to render that opinion?
- Should another, more appropriate, consultant have been requested?
- Who wrote the consultation note? *Did someone other than the attending physician write it? Does the note reflect that the attending physician reviewed and approved the findings of the intern, resident, or fellow with an additional signature at the bottom of the note?*
- What were the consultant's findings?

- Were the consultant's findings different from findings of the other treating physicians?
- Were the consultant's findings something the requesting physician should have discovered, had he or she exercised appropriate care in the history or physical examination?
- What further diagnostic tests or therapies did the consultant suggest?
- Did the consultant write orders in the chart? *Ordinarily, the consultant does not write orders in the chart but makes suggestions for diagnosis and treatment. The admitting physician who requested the consultation is expected to do all the ordering. If there is an emergency, or if the consultant becomes the primary treating physician, then the consultant may write orders in the chart as a treating physician.*
- Did the requesting physician write orders in the card reflecting the consultant's suggestions? If not, why?
- Was there a delay in following the consultant's suggestions?
- Was there an indication in the chart that the requesting physician did not agree with the consultant's findings or suggestions for treatment?
- If the admitting physician didn't agree with the consultant, was this disagreement explained?
- Were there any other communications between the requesting physician and the consultant? *Phone calls? E-mails? Hallway conversations?*
- What was the nature and content of any *ex parte* consultations?
- Were any changes in the therapeutic or treatment plans made by the consultant?
- Were any changes in the therapeutic or treatment plans made by the requesting physician?
- If there were any changes, what was the cause of these changes?
- If there were any changes, were they appropriate?

CHAPTER 16

Anesthesia Note

Q

What is an anesthesia note?

A

The *anesthesia note* is not only a recording of the interaction of the anesthesiologist and his patient, but also a minute-to-minute recording of a patient's physiologic responses to anesthesia. (See example in Figure 16.1.)

Q

Who is the author of the anesthesia note?

A

Two types of professionals perform anesthesia and record anesthesia notes:

- Anesthesiologists
- Certified Registered Nurse Anesthetists (CRNAs)

Anesthesiologists are physicians (MD or DO) who specialize in the practice of anesthesia. CRNAs are registered nurses who are specially trained to administer anesthesia. Both professionals perform many anesthesia services, including the following:

- Evaluating the patient for anesthesia pre- and postoperatively
- Providing various forms of anesthesia (e.g., generalized, localized, conscious sedation, and epidural anesthesia)
- Monitoring and supporting fluids, electrolytes, and ventilatory and metabolic functions during the surgical procedure

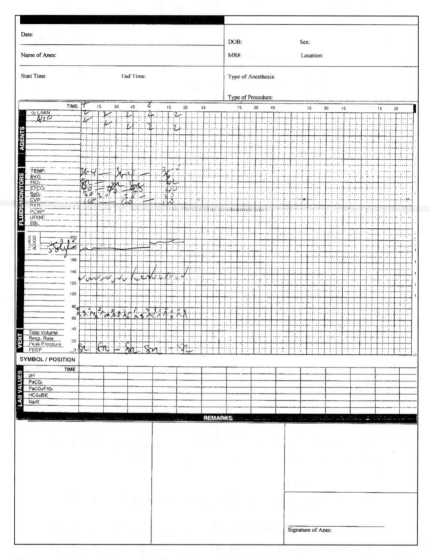

Figure 16.1   Example of an Anesthesia Note

 Q   **What is included in the anesthesia note?**

A   The anesthesia record should document the following information:

PREANESTHESIA EVALUATION

- Patient interview to assess medical and anesthetic histories
- Medication history

- Appropriate physical examination
- Review of objective diagnostic data (e.g., laboratory, ECG, and X-ray).
- Assignment of acetylsalicyclic acid (ASA) physical status
- Formulation of the anesthetic plan and discussion of the risks and benefits of the plan with the patient or the patient's legal representative

INTRAOPERATIVE/PROCEDURAL ANESTHESIA EVALUATION NOTE (TIME-BASED RECORD OF EVENTS)

- Immediate review prior to initiation of anesthetic procedures
- Reevaluation of the patient
- Check of equipment, drugs, and gas supply
- Monitoring of the patient (e.g., recording of vital signs, blood gas readings, cardiac output, etc.)
- Amounts of drugs and agents used, and times of administration
- The type and amounts of intravenous fluids used, including blood and blood products, and times of administration
- The technique(s) used
- Unusual events during the administration of anesthesia (e.g., difficulties in endotracheal intubation, insertion of central venous or arterial lines, difficulties with epidural punctures, sudden drops in blood pressure or oxygenation, etc.)
- The status of the patient at the conclusion of anesthesia

POSTANESTHESIA EVALUATION

- Patient evaluation on admission and discharge from the postanesthesia care unit
- A time-based record of vital signs and level of consciousness
- A time-based record of the drugs administered, their dosage, and route of administration
- Type and amounts of intravenous fluids administered, including blood and blood products
- Any unusual events, including postanesthesia or postprocedural complications
- Postanesthesia visits

Q   **What should be asked about the anesthesia note?**

- Who performed the anesthesia?

- What type of technique was used (e.g., general endotracheal, spinal, epidural, local, etc.)?
- What were their qualifications to perform this type of anesthesia?
- If a resident or CRNA administered the anesthesia, who was responsible for overseeing it?
- Was the anesthesiologist experienced or certified in the technique?
- Was the attending physician in the room during the induction phase of anesthesia?
- Was the attending physician in the room during any intra-operative or postoperative emergency?
- Was the patient at high risk for anesthesia complications?
- What monitoring devices were used during the anesthesia (e.g., Swan-Ganz catheter, intra-arterial line, central venous pressure monitors, intracerebral pressure monitor, etc.)?
- Were any complications noted during the placement of the monitoring devices?
- Were any complications noted during the endotracheal intubation?
- How was patient oxygenation monitored (e.g., continuous pulse oximetry or intermittent arterial blood gases)?
- Were any automatic alarms in place for physiologic monitoring?
  - What type of alarms?
  - Where they properly maintained?
  - When were these monitoring devices last inspected?
  - Were there complaints about the performance of these machines in the past?
  - If there were complaints, who made them?
  - Who was responsible for maintenance?
- Did any of the alarms sound during the case?
- Were there any significant episodes of low blood pressure, oxygen desaturation, or bleeding?
- How were these episodes handled?
- What was done to correct any physiologic abnormalities?
- If there were any physiologic abnormalities, who was involved in handling them? Was another anesthesia attending called in? Another surgeon? A nurse anesthetist?
- Was the patient's recovery uncomplicated?

- Was the patient arousable after anesthesia?
- Could the endotracheal tube be removed immediately?
- Did the anesthesiologist perform a post-anesthesia examination?
- Were there any post-anesthesia events (e.g., seizures, vomiting, aspiration, cardiac or respiratory arrest, or surgical site bleeding)?
- If there were any post-anesthesia events, how were they handled?
- If there were any post-anesthesia events, who handled them (e.g., nurses, residents, or attending physicians)?

CHAPTER 17

Procedure Note

Q
A
What is a procedure note?

When a patient undergoes a procedure in the hospital, a description of the procedure is recorded in the medical chart. The *procedure note* (operative note) attends every intervention, from a radiological procedure to brain surgery.

Q
A
Who is the author of the procedure or operative note?

The physician who performs the procedure or operation writes the note in the chart or dictates that note immediately after the procedure. In academic institutions, an intern or resident who aided in the procedure will be delegated with the task of composing the note. In this instance, the writer of the note will identify the person who performed the procedure and those who assisted.

Q
A
What information does the procedure note contain?

The notes can be relatively short, anywhere from handwritten notes in the medical chart to more extensive multi-page, dictated, and typewritten notes. A simple procedure note for the bedside insertion of a subclavian intravenous catheter should include the following data:

- Time and date
- Name of procedure

- Location of procedure (e.g., bedside, radiology suite, or OR)
- Indication for procedure
- Patient's status before procedure
- Consent obtained
- Anesthesia used
- Technique used
- Equipment used (e.g., # 14 IV catheter with triple lumen)
- Status of patient after the procedure (i.e., how patient tolerated procedure)
- Any confirmatory testing results (e.g., chest X-ray)
- Name of physician performing the procedure
- Name of any physicians who assisted in the procedure

Q

A

What information does the operative note contain?

For more complicated surgical procedures, the notes are more extensive. The operative note should include the following information:

- Time and date of procedure
- Name of all physicians participating in the procedure (e.g., first and second surgeons, resident, interns, and medical students that "scrub in" on the case)
- Name of procedure (e.g., appendectomy)
- Preoperative diagnosis (e.g., appendicitis)
- Type of anesthesia used (e.g., local, epidural, or general)
- Patient positioning (e.g., supine, Trendelenburg, or lithotomy)
- Patient preparation (e.g., shaving, topical antiseptics, and sterile draping)
- Step-by-step description of operative procedure, including the location of incisions and intra-operative findings, and instruments, closing techniques, and bandages used
- Operative mishaps (e.g., excessive bleeding, inadvertent punctures, avulsions, or lacerations) and what was done to correct them
- Miscellaneous operative information (e.g., estimated blood loss, tourniquet time, aortic cross-clamp time, biopsy tissue handling and disposition, instrument and sponge count, etc.)
- Condition of patient after procedure
- Postoperative diagnosis

- Dictation date
- Surgeon's signature

Q   **What should be asked about procedure or operative notes?**

- Who performed the surgery?
- Who assisted in the surgery?
- Was informed consent obtained?
- Was the patient in a condition to give informed consent?
- What was the indication for surgery? *Did the indication coincide with condition or finding on the admission note?*
- Was it an appropriate indication?
- Where was the surgery performed (e.g., hospital OR, emergency department, hospital bedside, outpatient surgical center, intensive care unit, etc.)?
- Was the procedure performed in an appropriate setting?
- If the procedure wasn't performed in an appropriate setting, why not?
- Was the procedure elective or emergent?
- Were any special monitoring devices used (e.g., intracerebral pressure monitors, esophageal ultrasound, intraarterial pressure monitors, etc.)?
- Why were these special monitors used?
- Who placed these monitors (e.g., surgeon, anesthesiologist, nurse anesthetist, radiologist)?
- Who was responsible for monitoring these special devices?
- How and where were results from any special devices recorded?
- How was the patient transferred from gurney to surgical table?
- Was a patient "roller" used to transfer the patient? *Surprisingly, many injuries can occur during this transfer, including lacerations, skin abrasion, joint dislocations, and bone fractures.*
- How was the patient positioned during surgery? *Improper positioning during a long surgical procedure can result in skin and muscle necrosis, decubitus ulcers, neuropathies, and limb ischemia.*
- Was a tourniquet used?
- If a tourniquet was used, where was it positioned?

- If a tourniquet was used, how long was it inflated?
- Was the preoperative and postoperative diagnosis the same?
- If the pre- and postoperative diagnoses were not the same, why not?
- Did a change in diagnosis result in any harm to the patient or delay in procedure?
- Was a change in diagnosis due to poor preoperative investigation?
- Were there any surgical complications?
- If there were any surgical complications, what were they?
- If there were any surgical complications, were those complications a known risk for the procedure?
- If a complication arose that was not a known risk for the procedure, why did it happen?
- Who was responsible for any complications (e.g., first surgeon, assistant surgeon, resident, scrub nurse, OR tech, etc.)?
- Were there any mechanical malfunctions of operative or monitoring instruments?
- Was an instrument and sponge count performed? Was the instrument and/or sponge count correct?

CHAPTER 18

Discharge Summary

Q
A

What is a discharge summary?

The *discharge summary* is a document that reviews significant events that occurred during a hospitalization. The discharge summary provides important information to other caregivers and facilitates the continuity of care. By regulation, it is part of every medical chart of a living discharged patient.

Q
A

Who writes the discharge summary?

The physician who has provided the majority of care for the patient writes the discharge summary. In academic institutions, discharge summaries are often the province of the lowest-ranking member of the care team (i.e., the intern or resident).

Q
A

What does the discharge summary contain? (See Figure 18.1.)

To comply with the Joint Commission on Accreditation of Healthcare Organizations, the discharge summary should contain the following information:

- Reason for hospitalization. *A brief statement of the patient's chief complaint and history of the present illness.*
- Significant objective findings. *Pertinent results of laboratory tests, radiological exams, and pathological studies.*

St. Vincent's Hospital
Discharge Summary

Last Name:	First Name:	Middle Initial: E.	SS#: 100-00-0000
Doe	John		
Street Address: 100 Main Street	City: Metropolis	State: New York	Zip code: 115500
Admission Date: 6/14/04	Discharge Date: 6/24/04	Primary Physician: Dr. Patricia Smith	

Admitting Diagnosis:	Discharge Diagnosis:
Exacerbation of Asthma	Community Acquired Pneumonia Exacerbation of Asthma

Clinical Course:

The patient is a 45 y/o white male with a past medical history of asthma who arrived at the ER via ambulance on 6/14/04, with complaints of SOB x 4 days. The SOB was accompanied by fever, sore throat and thick green sputum production. There was no chest pain, palpitations, dizziness or syncope. The patient was taking his usual medications including, ADVAIR 50/500, Alupent Sulfate MDI, and oral prednisone 40 mg / day.

The physical exam was significant for wheezing and decreased breath sounds in both lung fields. There was no dullness to percussion or egophony. There was no JVD, ankle swelling or cyanosis. No leg pain, leg swelling, pleuritic chest pain or hemoptysis. The physical exam was otherwise unremarkable.

The patient was admitted to the floor and treated with intravenous ampicillin and gentamycin for three days, then switched to oral Zithromycin. Prednisone was increased to 80 mg per day and Alupent sulfate was given by nebulizer Q 4 hrs.

Pulmonary consultation was called. Consultant agreed that DX was CAP and Asthma and agreed with treatment regimen.

The patient slowly improved and prednisone and nebulizers were decreased accordingly.

Repeat chest X-ray after 7 days demonstrated resolution of pulmonary infiltrate.

The patient's exercise capacity improved and he was able to ambulate more than 200 yrds without stopping.

Patient was discharged to home on 6/24/04.

Tests / Procedures:
- Chest x-ray: left lower lobe infiltrate c/w bacterial pneumonia. Repeat chest X-ray on 6/21/04 demonstrated resolution of infiltrate.
- EKG: NSR at 80, no ischemia
- CBC: WBC 22,000, with increased bands, H/H wnl
- Sputum gram stain: gram positive cocci in sheets
- Sputum Culture: oral pharyngeal flora
- Blood cultures: negative x 3

Figure 18.1   Discharge Summary

Medications on Discharge: • Prednisone: 10 mg / day PO, taper as directed • Advair 500/50 BID • Alupent MDI : as needed		
Follow Up Instructions: • Follow up with Dr. Patricia Smith (Pulmonology) in one week. • Return to ED for worsening SOB, Cough or fever.		
Physician's Name: (print)	**Physician's Signature:**	**Date:**

- Treatments rendered. *A review of any treatment or therapies that the patient received during the hospitalization; this includes medical, surgical, radiologic, pharmacologic, and rehabilitative treatments, among others.*
- Diagnoses. All relevant diagnoses.
- Patient's condition on discharge. *A summary clearly stating the patient's condition in measurable terms. Statements such as "improved" are vague and will not help the next physician or facility to judge any changes in the patient's condition.*
- Instructions to patient and family. *Instructions given to patient, patient's family, or other caregiver relative to physical activity, medications, diet, and follow-up care.*
- Signature of attending physician.

Q **What should be asked about the discharge summary?**

- Was the discharge summary completed by the attending physician or by an intern or resident?
- Does it mention tests, findings, or diagnoses not found in the medical chart? *Reviewing the discharge summary is a method of double checking that the medical record is complete. Tests, procedures, diagnoses, or incidents mentioned in the discharge summary should be found in the medical record, and vice versa.*
- Were all the prescriptions mentioned in the discharge summary actually given to the patient on discharge?
- Were any instructions given to the patient regarding recommended follow-up tests or treatments?

- Were clear instructions given to the patient about following up with the attending physician or other health care provider? Did this include a time and date? Was a specific provider or clinic mentioned? Was an appointment made for the patient?
- Was the discharge summary signed?
- Were specific instructions given to the patient about what to do after discharge if there are complications from the illness, injury, or surgical wounds (e.g., phone the physician immediately, return to the hospital's emergency department, or call an ambulance)?

CHAPTER 19

Radiology Report

Q **What is a radiology report?**

A The *radiology report,* or imaging report, describes the findings on a particular imaging study (e.g., X-rays, sonograms, radionuclear scans, CTs, or MRIs). The report is typically dictated, typed, and appended to the chart after 12–72 hours. When rare emergent situations demand it, the radiologist may write a note in the chart.

Q **Who writes the radiology report?**

A The radiology report is produced by the radiologist who "reads" the imaging study. This may not be the same radiologist who performed or supervised the imaging study. The author of the radiology report may not be the same radiologist who gave the "wet read" to the ED or surgical suite. A "wet read" is a reading done by a radiologist on an emergent basis. These "wet readings" are often given verbally by the radiologist. When radiologists do a "wet read," they do not have the benefit of a review of previous X-rays, nor can they refer the image to a radiologist more skilled at the interpretation of those types of imaging studies.

Q
A

What should the radiology report contain?

The radiology report should contain the following information:

- Date of procedure
- Date of report
- Name of procedure (e.g., anterior-posterior chest X-ray)
- Name of patient and medical record number of patient
- Description of type of X-ray technique (e.g., AP view of the upright chest)
- Notification of review of previous X-rays, if available
- Description of anatomy found in the radiograph. *This is the description or "findings" of the radiologist. These findings are significant positives and negatives of the exam: for example, "the heart silhouette is normal in contour without signs of enlargement, there is no indication of pleural effusions." The description also should state what is not included in the radiograph (e.g., lateral radiograph of cervical spine, including C1-C6. C7 is not visualized). These are often referred to as "study limitations."*
- Radiological diagnosis (e.g., transverse fracture of distal femur)
- Recommendations (e.g., repeat CT in 24 hours, or follow up chest X-ray in 3 months)
- Notifications. *In the event that radiograph demonstrates a dangerous or emergency situation, such as a pneumothorax, air in the biliary system, aortic aneurysm, or cervical spine fracture, the radiologist is obligated to notify the treating physician.*

Q

What should be asked about the radiology report?

- When was the X-ray ordered?
- When was the exam performed?
- Was the examination performed the examination that was requested by the physician? Was there a reason for any discrepancy?
- When was the X-ray read by the attending radiologist? Was it read by an ED physician, surgeon, radiology resident, or other physician in training?
- Was there an unusual delay in the reading? *Acceptable reading times vary depending on the type of exam and condition of the patient.*

- Were previous X-rays available?
- Did the radiologist report that the new X-ray examination was compared to previous X-rays?
- Was an interval change noted?
- Were any emergent conditions identified on the X-ray?
- Did the radiologist attempt to notify the ordering physician of the emergent condition? If so, did the radiologist report who was notified?
- Were further studies suggested? If so, were those studies ordered by the physician?
- Does the medical chart indicate that the physician read the X-ray report?
- Did the results of the report prompt appropriate action by the ordering physician (e.g., request confirmatory radiological tests, order other diagnostic tests, call a consultant, etc.)?

CHAPTER 20

Laboratory and Pathology Reports

Q
A

What are laboratory and pathology reports?

Laboratory and pathology reports are the recordings of clinical data that can be obtained from clinical laboratories. These data are derived from the clinical, chemical, or physical testing of human tissues or fluids. These reports come from many laboratories that are controlled or supervised by the pathology department. Laboratories that may report data to the physician and be attached to the medical chart include hematology, serology, bacteriology, toxicology, cytology, etc.

Q
A

Who creates laboratory and pathology reports?

In a community hospital, the hospital pathologist oversees not only tissue diagnosis from surgical biopsies and the results of autopsies, but also all analysis of other bodily fluids, such as blood, serum, and urine. This means, in the community hospital, the hospital pathologist is responsible for all of the laboratory services in the hospital. In larger university hospitals and academic centers, the lab services are overseen by nonphysician doctors of pathology, chemistry, or biochemistry.

The director of the laboratory employs and oversees the work of various laboratory technicians, cytologists, and lesser-skilled workers. These employees prepare and process samples, calibrate analyzers, and perform microscopic analysis of tissues and cultures.

Q   **Who writes the pathology report?**

A   Interpreting the results of pathology testing is the responsibility of the head pathologist, but is often performed by technicians, or by machines that technicians have maintained. Therefore, while the hospital pathologist may not have directly written a particular report or reviewed the output of an automated blood analyser, he or she is responsible for the accuracy and reproducibility of those results.

Q   **What is contained in laboratory and pathology reports?**

A   The following information is contained in laboratory and pathology reports:

- Surgical biopsy results
- Cytologic examination of cervical smears, blood, urine, cerebrospinal fluid (CSF), and other bodily fluids
- Chemical analysis of blood, cerebral spinal fluid, urine, etc.
- Microscopic analysis of cellular constituents of blood, CSF, urine, etc. (i.e., complete blood count)
- Toxicology screening
- DNA analysis

For the most part, these reports are computer generated and are entered into the hospital chart daily. Laboratory results that indicate an emergent condition (panic values) are reported to the ordering physician by the pathologist or one of his employees as soon as they are known.

Q   **What should be asked about laboratory and pathology reports?**

- When were the samples sent?
- When were the samples examined?
- When were "panic values" known by the laboratory staff?
- When were "panic values" reported to the ordering physician?
- To whom were the "panic values" reported?
- Who read the Pap smear? Pathologist? Cytologist?
- What is the procedure for "abnormal" Pap smears?

- Is there a published policy and procedure for "abnormal" Pap smears?
- Are "abnormal" Pap smears "over read" by one or more of the pathologists?
- What is the procedure for handling "abnormal" tissue biopsies?
- Are all "abnormal" tissue biopsies subject to examination and consensus of group pathologists, or are they read by only one pathologist?
- Did the treating physician acknowledge reading the report?
- Did the treating physician appropriately respond to the results of the report (i.e., change diagnostic or therapeutic plan to deal with the result)?
- If there was no change in the diagnostic or therapeutic plan, was an explanation given?
- What are the credentials of the pathologist reading the tissue biopsy? *Is the pathologist a dermatopathologist or neuropathologist? Some tissues are best read by specialists in that field of pathology.*

CHAPTER 21

Autopsy Report

Q
A

What is an autopsy report?

An *autopsy report* is a recording of a postmortem examination of a patient. The report is usually typed and may include toxicology reports, X-ray reports, histology reports, and photographs of autopsy findings. The autopsy report may be as brief as one typed page, or may run 8–12 typed pages.

Q
A

Who writes the autopsy report?

The autopsy report is written by the pathologist responsible for the postmortem examination. This pathologist is typically employed by a hospital. However, the Medical Examiner of the municipality will perform the autopsy in the case of an unexplained death or a death that occurs outside the hospital. When there is a suspicion of malpractice and the descendants are concerned about the objectivity of the hospital's pathologist, sometimes the next-of-kin will pay for an autopsy to be performed by an independent pathologist not affiliated with the local hospital.

Q
A

What information is included in the autopsy report?

Not all autopsies are the same. An autopsy that examines every tissue minutely and performs every test available would be very time-consuming and very expensive. Autopsies are not reimbursed under typical insurance plans, nor are they covered under Medicare or Medicaid. Pathologists are either employees of the hospital or are self-employed. As a result, pathologists are pressured to be as efficient as possible in performing their nonreimbursed autopsies. To this end, the pathologist makes an educated guess as to the cause of death. Then the pathologist tailors the autopsy to concentrate on the tissues or organ system involved. Therefore, an autopsy of a person with a known brain tumor will be different from the autopsy of a person with a known cardiac condition.

The typical autopsy report contains the following information:

- Name of patient
- Date of birth
- Date of death
- Date of autopsy
- Medical record number
- Autopsy report number
- Name of examining pathologist
- Names of others assisting in the autopsy (i.e., pathologists, residents, technicians, etc.)
- Inventory of personal effects
- Name of person(s) who identified the body
- Medical history
- External examination of the body
- Internal examination of the body (including the inspection and examination of each major organ of the body)
- Microscopic examination of tissues
- Toxicologic examination of blood, urine, and tissues (if called for by circumstances or ordered by physician or medical examiner)
- Radiologic examinations
- Microbiologic examination and cultures of blood or other bodily tissues
- Cause of death (e.g., myocardial infarction, cerebral hemorrhage, etc.)
- Manner of death (e.g., homicide, suicide, accidental, and "natural causes")

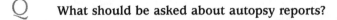

What should be asked about autopsy reports?

A   A learned pathologist, experienced in forensic examination of medical charts, once suggested that when examining an autopsy report, one should not look at what is in the report, but, rather, one should look for what is excluded from the report. The reviewer of the medical chart must keep in mind that pathologists are employed by the hospital, and, while they are honest and dedicated seekers of truth for the most part, occasionally some do succumb to pressure from their employers. For example, let's say an autopsy is performed on a patient who died suddenly two days after surgery. The true cause of death may be from a suture line on the bowel that has dehisced. The possible causes of this bad outcome include surgical error, bowel ischemia, mesenteric arterial thrombosis, pulmonary embolism, myocardial infarction, or stroke. The pathologist could attribute the cause of death to any one of these. If he chooses surgical error as the cause of death, it could result in a massive malpractice suit against both the hospital and the surgeon. For a pathologist who is more concerned with continued employment than the truth, omitting a full examination of the bowel on his autopsy report often is seen as a workable compromise. Similarly, in a case of a potential medication overdose, the less-than-scrupulous pathologist may "forget" to perform a toxicology screen during the autopsy. Without evidence of the medication overdose in the toxicology screen, a malpractice case for medication error would be difficult to prosecute. Therefore, the seasoned reviewer would review the autopsy report and attempt to compare the alleged cause of death with the examinations on the autopsy report. Missing data should be noted on the chart and referred to the attorney for expert review.

Q   **What else should be asked about autopsy reports?**

- Who performed the autopsy? *Was the autopsy performed by the hospital pathologist or a consulting pathologist?*
- Who else was present at the autopsy (e.g., pathologists, residents, technicians, or police)?
- Who requested the autopsy? *Was the autopsy requested by the family, hospital, physician, or law enforcement? Did the family*

pay for the autopsy themselves? Why did the family request an autopsy? What were they looking for?

- Was the autopsy limited in any way? *Sometimes next-of-kin will only give permission for a limited autopsy. This may involve only postmortem biopsies and sampling of bodily fluids. From a forensic standpoint, these autopsies are useless for determining cause of death.*
- If the autopsy was limited, who placed the limitations on the autopsy?
- Were all the organs or organ systems examined?
- Was the cardiovascular system examined?
- Was the pulmonary system examined?
- Was the neurologic system examined (including an examination of the brain and meninges)?
- Was toxicology screening done?
- Were tissues examined microscopically?
- Were any special tests performed on the tissue? Why were these special tests performed? What was the pathologist looking for?
- Are all the test results that were ordered on the chart? *It may take months to receive the results of tests after the samples have been sent for examination.*
- Is the autopsy report finalized? *In some cases, the autopsy report will be prepared before all the test results have been received. Any findings on this report are preliminary. The finalized report should be sought out.*
- Has the report been signed by the pathologist who performed the autopsy or a supervising pathologist?
- Does the pathologist's determination of cause of death coincide with the suspected cause of death?
- Are the organ systems that were suspected in the cause of death fully examined?

CHAPTER 22

Nursing Notes

Q
A

What are nursing notes?

Nursing notes constitute a large portion of each medical chart. The *nursing notes* should reflect, at their best, an hour-to-hour assessment of the patient's physical and mental condition, his responses to therapy, and relevant communications with the health care team.

Q
A

Who creates nursing notes?

The nursing notes that appear in a patient's chart are written by the team of nurses who care for the patient. During a single 24-hour period, a minimum of three nurses will enter notes on the patient's chart. If the patient undergoes any therapy or diagnostic testing, it is likely that a different nurse will enter notes on the chart. For example, if the patient undergoes cardiac stress testing or an MRI, nurses attached to those units will enter notes. If the patient is transferred between units (e.g., from the intensive care unit to the medical ward), nurses from each unit will make observations and assessments and write them in the chart. If any procedure is done on the patient (e.g., a bedside surgical procedure or resuscitation), the note may not be written by the nurse who usually cares for the patient, but by a nurse attached to the surgical or resuscitation team.

Q

A

How are nursing notes organized?

Like the physician progress notes, nursing notes should have a standard format. There are many standardized formats for nursing notes. Regardless of the system of documentation that is used, the nursing note should contain the following elements:

- Assessment. *The critical observing of the client for signs and symptoms that may indicate actual or potential problems. These signs and symptoms include subjective patient complaints and objective findings from physical examination and test results.*
- Planning. *The development of a plan of care directed at preventing, minimizing, or resolving identified client problems or issues.*
- Implementation. *The utilization of the plan of care that has been developed. This includes the specific actions that the nurse needs to take to activate that plan.*
- Evaluation. *The determination of whether the plan of care was effective in preventing, minimizing, or resolving identified problems.*

Q

A

What does the nursing note contain?

The nursing note should contain the following information:

- Date and time
  - The date and time of when the nursing note was written
  - The date and time of when activities or events occurred

- Physical assessment
  - Vital signs
  - General assessment
    - Glasses? Dentures? Hearing aids? Is there anything that the caretakers need to be aware of to properly care for this patient?

  - Heart exam
  - Lung exam
  - Abdominal exam
  - Neurologic exam
  - Skin

- Is the skin intact?
- Is there any sign of skin breakdowns or decubitus ulcers?
- Are there sutures? Surgical wounds? Dressings?

- Extremities
  - Are all four extremities without defect?
  - Amputations
  - Paresis

- Record of abnormal physical findings
  - Name of person to whom abnormal findings were reported
  - Date and time of report of abnormal findings
  - Record of intervention to improve or treat abnormality
  - Patient response to the intervention

- Patient inputs
  - Dietary or nutritional assessment
  - Patient height
  - Patient weights taken daily and compared with admission weight
  - What has the patient eaten?
  - What has the patient had to drink?

- Patient outputs
  - Urine output
  - Drainage from chest tubes or wound drains
  - Stool

- Patient comfort
  - Is the patient in pain?
  - What is the cause?
  - What can be done to decrease the pain (e.g., positioning and analgesic medication)?

- Psychosocial assessment
  - Assessment of patient's mood
  - Assessment of the patient's level of understanding of his disease state
  - Assessment of patient's ability to care for himself or herself

- Communications
  - Record of time, date, and substance of contact with patient's next-of-kin
  - Record of time, date, and substance of contact with physicians in care team
  - Record of time, date, and substance of any orders given by physicians in the care team
  - Record of time, date, and substance of any conversation with physicians or other members of the health care team where information about the patient's condition was discussed or a request for patient evaluation was made
- Medications
  - The name of the medication, dose, timing, and route of administration
  - Any reason for not administering the ordered medication
  - Any reason for altering the dosage or timing of the medication
  - Any adverse reactions to the medication
- Patient interventions
  - There should be a record of what therapies or diagnostic tests were ordered. The record should include the following information:
    - Which tests, therapies, or procedures the patient underwent
    - A record of when they occurred
    - A record of the patient's response
- Patient safety
  - Patient's ability to ambulate or transfer
  - The distance that the patient can ambulate safely
  - Need for assistance in ambulation or transfer
  - Need for assistive devices for ambulation or transfer (e.g., walker, cane, leg brace, transfer board, etc.)
  - Use and position of bed side rails
  - Patient instruction on the use of call bell and the fact that the call bell was placed within the patient's reach
  - Need for restraints. Type of restraints. Duration of need for restraints.
  - Need for any special monitoring (e.g., risk of wandering or elopement)

- Interpreters
  - Ability of patient to understand spoken and written English
  - Ability of patient to repeat instructions in his or her own words
  - Assessment of need for translation services
  - Name of person who provided translation services

WHAT SHOULD BE ASKED ABOUT THE NURSING NOTES?

- Who wrote the note? *Is the name of the nurse legible? Can the name be deduced using a copy of the nursing schedule?*
- What are the qualifications of the nurse writing the note? *The nurse's signature should be followed by his or her credentials. There is a wide spectrum of certifications in the nursing profession. A nurse's training may range from two to six years. Knowing the credentials of the nurse, as well as his or her level of experience, helps to give credibility to his or her observations.*
- When was the note written? *Is the time and date clear? Are time entries on the chart written in military time format (now recommended as the standard format)? Can AM and PM times be clearly distinguished? Are the notes in a clear chronological order?*
- Do the notes adequately reflect the condition of the patient at the time they are written? *While the nursing notes, like the physician progress notes, tend to be formulaic and standardized, they should reflect any changes in the patient's condition. The notes should not only record unstable vital signs, but also record more data about the changing condition and the nurse's effort to stabilize them, especially the nurse's communications with other members of the health care team and with the family.*
- Do the nurse's notes record a patient complaint or dangerous condition that is not addressed subsequently in the notes? *When a nurse notices a condition that would alter the patient's safety or comfort, he or she is obliged to act quickly to remedy the situation. The reviewer should carefully read the nurse's notes looking for responses to dangerous conditions that arose. Are these responses adequate? Is the condition adequately resolved?*
- Do the nursing notes conflict with the physician's notes regarding the patient's condition? *Any conflict between the assessments of two members of the health care team should be noted in the review and investigated further. A conflict in assessment does not imply an attempt*

to hide information or even negligence, but may reflect a rapidly chang-
ing medical condition or differences in abilities and experience of the
people doing the assessing.

- Do the nursing notes correspond with the physician notes regarding bedside procedures, tests, and physician assessments? *While some tests and bedside procedures can occur without the patient's nurse's awareness of this, in general, the nurse's notes record all tests and pro-cedures. This is especially true if the patient is unstable, the bedside test is invasive or complicated, or the patient is required to leave the nursing floor for a test.*

- Is there evidence of communications by physicians to nurses (found in the physician progress note, for example) that do not appear in the nursing note?

- Is there evidence of requests by nurses to physicians for patient eval-uation that are not responded to? *When are these recorded? How many times did the nurse call? Did the nurse indicate the condition of the patient or why the evaluation was needed? When, if ever, did the physician respond?*

- Were the medications that were ordered by the physician adminis-tered by the nurse? *Was the medication administered to the patient? Was there a time difference between the order and the administration? Was there an unnecessary delay in the administration of a critical medi-cation? If there was, what was the cause of the delay? Did this delay result in harm to the patient?*

- Were the medications that were ordered by the physician adminis-tered by the nurse in the dosage, timing, and route ordered by the physician? *One should compare the physician's order form with the nurse's administration record. Are there any translation errors in the names of the medication or in the decimal points in the dosages? Are there any errors in the route of administration (e.g., an intramuscular medication given as an intravenous medication)?*

- Was the nurse given discretion in the use of the medication? *In some situations, physicians may order medication to be given at the discretion of the nurse. These medications include analgesics such as ibuprofen, acetaminophen, or morphine sulfate (e.g., "Morphine Sulfate 2-10 mg sc for pain prn Q 4 hours."). Insulin may also be given according to an agreed upon "sliding scale." Here, the physician outlines the parameters of insulin administration in response to the results of regular blood glu-cose measurements. Were the physician orders clear as to the appropri-ate medication, dose, timing, and route? Was the physician clear in his* orders as to the appropriate indications for the use of the medications? Were instructions given by the physician about when he should be called for clarification or intervention (e.g., "notify MD if the blood glucose rises above 500 mg/ dl")?

- Was the nurse given orders to notify the physician when there are changes in the patient's condition? Were specific parameters given like, "notify MD if the oxygen saturation drops below 80%" or "Notify MD if the systolic blood pressure rises above 180 mmHg?" Were these orders followed?

- Was the patient able to communicate with nurses? Could the patient speak with nurses and express his needs? If not, how was this overcome? Was a communication device such as a signboard used? Was the patient able to use the nurse call button? Do the nurse's notes reflect that instructions on the use of the call button were given and that it was placed within reach of the patient?

- Were physician orders given for the use of restraints? What were the indications for the use of restraints? Are the restraints removed after the indications for their use no longer exist? Do the nurse's notes record frequent observation of the patient in restraints and their safety?

- Were bed rails used? Bed rails are a safety device used to keep patients from falling out of bed. Those at risk for falling out of bed are elderly patients, demented patients, patients obtunded from medications, and patients confused from injury or infection. These conditions should prompt the nurse to put up the bed rails. The identified "at risk" condition and the fact that the bed rails have been "put up" should be noted in the chart. For some confused patients, putting up the bed rails only serves as a challenge, and they may attempt to leave the bed by climbing over the rails. This places the patient at greater risk for fall and injury than not having the rails up at all. For patients like these, restraints are indicated. Has the patient attempted to leave the bed over the rails in the past? Have restraints been requested? Have the physicians ordered them? Are the nurse's observations more frequent because the patient is in restraints?

- Are any conflicts noted in the nursing notes? The hospital environment can be stressful; at times, these stresses appear in the nurse's notes. This type of entry is discouraged by the hospital's risk manager for obvious reasons. The reviewer should note and report all mentions of the following conflicts:
  - Nurse to nurse conflicts
  - Nurse to patient-family conflicts

- Nurse to physician conflicts
- Physician to patient-family conflicts
- Complaints about understaffing of nurses or nurse's aides
- Complaints about mandatory overtime
- Complaints about overwhelming patient assignments
- Conflict between a nurse's training and experience and her present assignment (e.g., putting a nurse experienced in labor and delivery to work in the emergency department or the intensive care unit)

CHAPTER 23

Medical Policies

Q
A
What is a medical policy?

A *medical policy* is a high-level, overall plan that describes the general goals of the institution and sets forth the acceptable actions in a particular medical setting.

Q
A
Who writes medical policies?

The medical policy is written by a person or people who are aware of the safest, most effective way to accomplish a particular action in a medical setting, whether that is treating a myocardial infarction in the emergency department or sterilizing surgical equipment in the operative suite. These knowledgeable people include the chiefs of departments, risk managers, and, in larger institutions, a policy committee. In an office or small clinic, the responsibility for developing policies usually falls to the most senior and experienced physician.

Q
A
Why do they exist?

Medical policies exist in order to guide medical decision making and to achieve the safest, most effective way of dealing with a medical situation. Further, many medical facilities have policies to satisfy regulatory mandates from federal, state, and private insurance plans (e.g., CMS, Joint Commission, NCQA, HMOs, etc.).

Q   **What do medical policies contain?**

A   Medical policies contain the following information:

- Date of implementation
- Date of expiration
- Statement of purpose
- Goals of policy
- Procedures for complying with policies
- Definitions
- Authorizing signature

Q   **How are medical policies used in litigation?**

A   While policies are used by hospitals and physician practices to identify and enforce the perceived best method for handling medical situations, in the legal setting, policies are used to establish the medical "standard of care."

Q   **How are medical policies used to establish a "standard of care?"**

A   For most medical malpractice actions, the ability to define the "standard of care" and to prove that the "standard of care" has been breached is the cornerstone of the case. Although legal definitions of the "standard of care" abound (and differ from state to state), applying these definitions to specific cases can prove a daunting task, as the definition is undermined by subjectivism. Therefore, if a hospital uses a policy to identify the best method of accomplishing a medical therapy, this may be considered, by some, the "standard of care" for that locality. Further, deviations from these policies may be construed as negligent acts.

In a malpractice setting, the attorneys on both sides will commonly request copies of any policies the medical facility has created that relate to the alleged negligent act.

The courts have held that hospital policies can be used to prove the "standard to care." For example, in the case of *Moyer v. Reynolds,*[1] an ED physician examined the plaintiff, a 33-year-old woman, who complained of chest pain and shortness of breath. An abnormal cardiogram was misinterpreted by the ED physician as nonsignificant. The hospital policy stated that abnormal electrocardiograms needed to be reviewed by a cardiologist

[1]780 So. 2d 205 (Fla. 2001).

before the patient could be discharged. The patient was discharged before a cardiologist had a chance to look at the ECG and died at home a few hours later. An autopsy confirmed a death by myocardial infarction. In the first trial of this incident, the hospital policies were not introduced into evidence, and the jury found for the defendant. However, on appeal, the reviewing court held that the hospital's policies and procedures do provide evidence of the "standard of care." They noted that there was a possibility that if the ED physician had complied with the policy in effect, then the on-call cardiologist would have been consulted and the patient could have survived the heart attack. Since Florida courts allow a claimant in a medical malpractice action "to establish that the health care provider breached his or her own rule of practice or violated an industry standard as evidence of the standard of care," the trial court's failure to allow the cardiologist's testimony regarding the hospital policies required that the jury's verdict be reversed.

The Georgia court of appeals extended the influence of hospital policies by holding, in *Byrd v. Medical Center of Central Georgia, Inc.*,[2] that a physician not only could be considered negligent for failing to follow established department guidelines, but also could be considered negligent for not knowing that the guidelines existed. Ignorance is not an excuse in these situations.

Q   **What should be asked about hospital, clinic, or physician office policies?**

- Does a policy manual exist?
- Does the manual's policy cover the situation in the alleged negligence?
- Who wrote the policy? *If a chief of department is alleged to have acted negligently and is in deviation of a policy that he or she authored, the policy may be more dispositive in the establishment of the standard of care.*
- When was the medical policy last updated? *Old and neglected policy manuals can be discredited if the policy doesn't reflect current thinking on the matter at hand.*
- Was the policy updated immediately after the incident in question? Has the policy been gratuitously changed to support the actions of the physician or nurse defendant?

---

[2]574 S.E.2d 326 (Ga. 2002).

CHAPTER 24

Incident Reports

Incident reports are not typically part of the medical record nor are they likely to be mentioned in the medical record. However, if they can be produced during discovery, incident reports can be very helpful to the medical chart reviewer as they may contain revealing information that identifies new witnesses and opens new avenues of discovery. The data contained in the incident report may help to more fully explain the chain of events that led to the adverse outcome or negligence.

What is an incident report?

An *incident report* (also called an unusual occurrence report) is a document that contains the results of an investigation about an adverse event within the hospital. Most hospitals require the nursing staff to fill out incident reports when a problem in medical care delivery has occurred. The problems in incident reports involve serious deviations from accepted clinical practice that resulted, or could have resulted, in an injured patient. These reports are meant to be nonjudgmental, factual reports of the problem and its consequences. (See an example of an incident report in Figure 24.1.)

Who is the author of an incident report?

The manager or director of the involved departments writes the incident report. These directors are responsible for carrying out the investigation, including interviewing all the participants and

Acme Hospital
Incident Report

☐ Not Part of the Medical Record
☐ For Quality Assurance Purposes Only

Subject's Name: _____
Ward: _____
Date: _____
Reported by: _____

☐ Inpt.   ☐ Outpt.   ☐ Visitor   ☐ Employee   ☐ Other   Birthdate ☐☐ ☐☐ ☐☐☐☐   Sex: ☐ Male   ☐ Female

OCCURRENCE DATA	FOR RM USE ONLY	Severity Index:	Reportable to: DOH ☐ Yes ☐ No
Date ||||| Time |||| ☐ AM ☐ PM		☐ Level I ☐ Level III ☐ Level II ☐ Level IV	MEDWATCH ☐ Yes ☐ No Product/Drug Lot No.: _____

OCCURRENCE LOCATION

☐ Amb. Surgery   ☐ Detoxification   ☐ Grounds/Parking Lot   ☐ Nuclear Medicine   ☐ Physical Therapy   ☐ Step Down Unit
☐ Cardiac Cath.   ☐ Dialysis   ☐ Home Care   ☐ Nursery   ☐ Psychiatry   ☐ Surgery
☐ Clinic   ☐ Emergency Dept.   ☐ Labor & Delivery   ☐ OB/GYN   ☐ Radiation Therapy   ☐ Telemetry
☐ Critical Care   ☐ Extended Care   ☐ Laboratory   ☐ Operating Room   ☐ Radiology   ☐ Transport
☐ Dentistry   ☐ Gen. Med./Surg.   ☐ Lobby/Common Area   ☐ PACU   ☐ Rehabilitation   ☐ Other _____
   ☐ Medicine   ☐ Pediatrics   ☐ Satellite Site

OCCURRENCE CATEGORY

Select one category (Oval) only: Under the Falls category, select one box in each section. For all other categories, you may select up to 2 boxes by marking them with numbers 1 and 2, indicating the primary and secondary nature of the occurrence.

FALLS ◯

OBSERVED   **ASSISTED**
☐ Yes   ☐ Yes
☐ No   ☐ No
LOCATION
☐ Patient's Bathroom
☐ Patient's Room
☐ Unit Hallway
☐ Other _____
ACTIVITY PRIOR TO FALL
☐ In Bed
☐ On Commode/Toilet
☐ In Chair/Wheelchair
☐ Standing/Walking
☐ In Tub/Shower
☐ On Stretcher/Table/Equipment
☐ Unknown
☐ Other _____
CAUSE
☐ Slipped/Tripped ☐ Weak/Collapse
☐ Unknown ☐ Other _____
FLOOR   **BED ALERT**
☐ Wet ☐ Dry   ☐ Y ☐ N ☐ N/A
SIDERAILS UP   **RESTRAINTS**
☐ Y ☐ N ☐ N/A   ☐ Y ☐ N ☐ N/A
ACTIVITY ORDERS: _____

PROCEDURE ◯ **or TEST** ◯
or TREATMENT ◯
☐ Allergic/Adverse reaction
☐ Break in sterile technique
☐ Cancellation
☐ Contamination
☐ Delay/Failure to review results
☐ Delay in performance/Results
☐ Error in performance/Results
☐ Delay/Error in reporting results
☐ Equipment failure/Malfunction
☐ Foreign body
☐ Implant failure
☐ Improper/Lack of consent
☐ Incorrect OR count
☐ Intolerance
☐ Lack of adequate monitoring
☐ Lost/Mishandled specimen
☐ Not ordered
☐ Ordered, not done
☐ Patient refusal
☐ Trauma from/Complication of
☐ Wrong patient/Site
☐ Wrong procedure/Test/Treatment
☐ Other _____

MEDICATION ◯ **or BLOOD** ◯ **or IV** ◯
☐ Allergic/Adverse reaction   ☐ Omission
☐ Contaminated/Outdated   ☐ Patient refusal
☐ Delay in administration   ☐ Pharmacy related
☐ Discontinued   ☐ Wrong dose
☐ Discontinued by patient   ☐ Wrong flow rate
☐ Duplicated   ☐ Wrong medication
☐ Equipment failure/Malfunction   ☐ Wrong patient
☐ Improper/Lack of consent   ☐ Wrong route
☐ Incorrect narcotic count   ☐ Wrong solution
☐ Infiltration   ☐ Wrong time
☐ Mislabeled   ☐ Other _____

Was a transcription error involved?   ☐ Yes   ☐ No

MISCELLANEOUS ◯
☐ Assault/Altercation   ☐ Power failure
☐ Attempt suicide/Suicide   ☐ Pt./Family/Visitor complaint
☐ Burns   ☐ Patient interference
☐ Elopement   ☐ Property loss/Damage
☐ Fire   ☐ Self-extubation
☐ Food/Beverage related   ☐ Self-inflicted injury
☐ Left AMA   ☐ Spill/Leak
☐ Left BT/Left WCT   ☐ Unauthorized drugs/Smoking
☐ Needlestick   ☐ Other

ACCOUNT OF OCCURRENCE (Print) _____

Printed Name	Signature	Title	Ext.	Date

OUTCOME
☐ Abrasion/Blister/Skin tear   ☐ Burn/Scald   ☐ Hemorrhage   ☐ Reaction/Toxic effect
☐ Aggravated pre-exist. condition   ☐ Code/Arrest   ☐ Infection   ☐ Reddened
☐ Aspiration/Anoxia   ☐ Death   ☐ Laceration   ☐ Sprain/Strain
☐ Bruise/Ecchymosis/Hematoma   ☐ Dental injury   ☐ Neurologic injury   ☐ Swelling/Phlebitis
   ☐ Fracture/Dislocation   ☐ No injury   ☐ Other _____

CHANGE IN DISPOSITION
☐ None/Unknown
☐ Extended hospital stay
☐ Unplanned return to OR
☐ Transferred to higher level of care
☐ Transferred to tertiary care facility

FOLLOW-UP   MD Called? ☐ Yes ☐ No ☐ N/A   Radiologic Study Ordered? ☐ Yes ☐ No ☐ N/A
Occurrence Diagnosis _____   Treatment _____
Physician/Supervisor Name _____   Signature _____   Date _____

Figure 24.1   Example of an Incident Report

examining of what records and other evidence are available. These directors examine the impact on the patient, identify who participated in the event, and search for the event's causes.

What do the incident reports contain?

The incident report usually contains two complementary sections. These are the data entry form and investigates narrative report.

The *data entry form* is often preprinted and contains the basic patient identification data, demographic data, a checklist of different types of incidents (e.g., slip and fall, patient elopement, medication error, etc.), and a space for written comments (see Figure 24.1). The aim of this is to provide a short form of information for data entry into a quality assurance database. This information will provide the grist for trend analysis, as well as prospective and retrospective quality-improvement research or quality-improvement programs.

The *investigator's narrative report* is an opportunity for the supervisor to further explain the events that led up to or caused the adverse event. This narrative report should include only factual information, results of interview of the parties involved, and a description of the consequences of the event. The report should not draw any conclusions, make any accusations, or place blame on any employee. However, this often happens. Chart reviewers should be alert for any suggestions of subjectivity in the report. This may suggest further witnesses or new avenues of investigation.

Why are incident reports created?

Incident reports are created for two reasons: compliance with Joint Commission standards and quality improvement programs.

In determining compliance with Joint Commission standards,[1] Joint Commission inspectors are now asking to see both the hospital's plan for complying with the quality assurance regulations and the minutes of the various hospital committees.

In an effort to improve the standard of care and clinical outcomes, the hospital employs quality assurance and peer review

---

[1] "An organization-wide Information Collection and Evaluation System (ICES) is developed and used to evaluate conditions in the environment of care." *Comprehensive Accreditation Manual for Hospitals, CAMH 1996:369.*

committees. It is the mission of a hospital quality assurance pro-gram and the legal duty of the quality assurance supervisor to identify and take the steps necessary to prevent recurring prob-lems with patient care. Incident report data are essential to this process.

Are incident reports discoverable?

Hospital administrators and risk managers maintain that the incident reports created by nurses and others in the hospital are not discoverable. They assert that these reports are created for the purpose of improving the quality of care. If the writers of these reports feel that the next person reading the report will be a plaintiff's attorney, the reports will likely lack the depth of data necessary to effect improvements in quality.

Reports created for the purpose of medical quality improve-ment are protected by statute. However, these statutes do not apply to administrative documents, especially those created by nonphysicians.

Incident reports are immune to discovery when the document is the product of a quality assurance or peer review committee or when the report is covered under the aegis of attorney-client privilege.

The source, as well as the purpose underlying the generation of an incident report, will determine whether such reports are subject to discovery. For example, when a quality assurance or peer review committee generates the incident report for the pur-pose of improving clinical outcomes, the report should be immune from discovery. Similarly, if an incident report is created at the request of the hospital's attorney for the purpose of defending the hospital against lawsuits, then the document is considered protected under the attorney-client privilege. In both these situations, a written hospital policy should reflect the clear purpose of the incident report.

When is the incident report discoverable?

An incident report may be discoverable under the following conditions:

- If the incident report was created at the behest of a hospital administrator for the purpose of statistical analysis or personnel evaluation, for example. *Discovery of this document would still be possible, even if the data were subsequently used by the hospital attorney or by the quality assurance committee.*

- If the existence of the report is mentioned, or its content discussed, in the medical chart. *The discovery would be allowable under the "incorporation by reference" rule. Incorporation by reference is the method of making one document of any kind become part of another separate document by referring to the former in the latter. Therefore, any mention of the incident report in the clinical chart makes the incident report part of the clinical chart. Similarly, if there is mention in the chart of a staff member giving testimony to investigators of an adverse incident, the testimony (often recorded in the incident report) becomes discoverable under the same incorporation by reference rule.*

- If a hospital is suspected of being liable in a lawsuit for a pattern of negligence, or if ongoing criminal misconduct continues to harm patients after events have afforded a clear-enough basis for quality assurance to see that something is going on and take action. *In this situation, the hospital's incident reports (or lack thereof) may be discoverable during an investigation of the hospital's quality assurance program.*[2]

- If the plaintiff has substantial need for the information contained in the incident report, yet is unable to get the same or similar information as is contained in the incident report without undue hardship. *In this situation, the courts have waived the immunity of these documents.*[3]

While the distinctions between discoverable and nondiscoverable seem clear-cut, there have been no consistent rulings by the courts. In fact, an increasing number of courts have allowed discovery of incident reports when the plaintiff can demonstrate a convincing need. Even insurers, third party payers, public health, federal, and state legislators have been exercising their fiduciary rights to examine the incident reports. Therefore, the medical reviewer should examine the chart and look for clues that may make this document discoverable.

[2]*Gess vs. U.S.*, 952 F. Supp. 1529 (M.D. Ala., 1996).

[3]*The Attorney–Client Privilege and work product doctrine.* 2nd edition, American Bar Association, pages 130–139.

The medical reviewer should seek the following in the clinical chart to aid in discovery of incident reports:

- Determine what is the facility's name for an incident report (e.g., unusual occurrence report, adverse event report, untoward event report, medical error report, etc.).
- Determine if there is any mention of the incident report in the clinical chart.
- Determine if there is mention in the clinical chart of testimony to an investigator or investigatory body by personnel involved in the incident. *For example, the courts have been unequivocal in ordering the production of witness statements where witnesses do not recollect events or substantial time has elapsed since the incident occurred.*[1]
- Determine whether the event was part of a pattern of similar events in the hospital, and obtain any studies done about them.

IF AN ADVERSE EVENT REPORT IS REVIEWED, THE FOLLOWING INFORMATION SHOULD BE SOUGHT:

- Names of all personnel involved in the adverse event
- Names of all departments involved
- Names of all personnel involved in the investigation of the event and generation of the incident report
- All notes taken during testimony and discussion of adverse incident
- Notes prepared by witnesses at the request of nurse managers or risk managers
- Reports prepared by agents of the defendant reflecting facts discovered during an on-site investigation or witness interviews
- Complete testimonies about the event from all interviewed personnel
- Any determination of liability, blame, or fault by the investigator or committee
- The nature of sanctions, training, preventative actions, or quality research that stem from this adverse event

Q   **What should be asked about an incident report?**

- Who authored the incident report?
- Is the author the manager or director of the department in which the incident occurred?
- If the author is other than the manager or director of the department in which the incident occurred, why is this?

---

[1] *The United States v. Murphy Cook and Company*, F.2d, F.D.R. 363, (E.D. Pa, 1971).

- What personnel are mentioned in the incident report?
- Are names mentioned that do not occur in the clinical record?
- Does the report indicate liability on the part of anyone?
- Does the report blame a device or lack thereof?
- Does the report implicate a lack of staffing as an issue?
- Does the report indicate that this is not the first time this event occurred?
- Are other incidents hinted at?
- Could there be other reports related to this patient or to members of the health care team?
- Does the report contradict events as recorded in the medical record?
- Does the incident report contradict events as recorded in depositions by witnesses?

CHAPTER 25

Medication Errors

INTRODUCTION

A *medication error* can be defined as any preventable event that may cause or lead to inappropriate medication use or patient harm while the medication is in the control of the health care professional, patient, or consumer.[1]

According to the 1991 Harvard Medical Practice Study, the leading cause of medical injury in hospitals is the misuse of drugs, accounting for 19.4% of injuries.[2] In fact, complications resulting from drug therapy or adverse drug reactions account for nearly one out of five adverse events that cause injury or death to patients each year.[3] These injuries are costly. For example, a 1997 study found that an adverse drug event is typically associated with a prolonged hospital stay and excess costs of around $2,000.[4] Patient injuries and increased cost are not the only issues. The Institute of Medicine estimates that preventable medication errors result in more than 7,000 deaths each year in hospitals alone and tens of thousands more in outpatient facilities.

---

[1]National Coordinating Council for Medication Error Reporting and Prevention.

[2]D. W. Bates et al., "Incidence of Adverse Drug Events and Potential Adverse Drug Events: Implications for Prevention," *JAMA*, 274(1), July 5, 1995, pp. 29–34.

[3]Research Activities, "System Changes May Reduce Hospital Medication Errors," *Am Health Syst Pharm*, 185(6), 1995, p. 3.

[4]D. C. Classen et al., "Adverse Drug Events in Hospitalized Patients," *JAMA*, 277(4), January 22/29, 1997, pp. 301–306.

This chapter will cover the process by which patients receive drugs in hospitals, from the physician order, to pharmacy filling, to nurse administration. The focus of this chapter will be on the areas where medication errors typically occur and how a reviewer can find evidence of these errors in the medical chart.

COMPONENTS OF APPROPRIATE DRUG ADMINISTRATION

The following are the five rights of proper drug administration:

- The right drug
- Administered by the right route
- At the right dose
- To the right patient
- At the right time

Drug orders are given millions of times per day, and a drug order requires little effort on the physician's part. The ease and the frequency of the drug administration process belies its complexity and the ease that errors can slip into the process. A single drug order may involve up to six professionals, three departments, and take several hours to complete. The drug name and dose may be transcribed three or four times before the drug is administered. The multiple steps and people involved in a single drug order predisposes the drug administration process to errors. In fact, the few hospitals that have studied incidence rates of adverse drug reactions have documented rates ranging from 2 to 7 per 100 admissions.[5,6,7,8]

Q   **Where do drug errors occur?**

A   A prospective study in 1995 of 4031 adult admissions found that most medication errors resulted from mistakes made at the ordering stage, but that many also occurred at the administration stage.[9]

---

[5]D. W. Bates et al., "Relationship Between Medication Errors and Adverse Drug Events," *J Gen Intern Med,* 10, 1995, pp. 199–205.

[6]D. J. Cullen et al., "The Incident Reporting System Does Not Detect Adverse Drug Events: A Problem for Quality Improvement," *Jt Comm J Qual Improv,* 21, 1995, pp. 541–548.

[7]D. J. Cullen et al., "Preventable Adverse Drug Events in Hospitalized Patients: A Comparative Study of Intensive Care and General Care Units," *Crit Care Med,* 25, 1997, pp. 1289–1297.

[8]D. C. Classen et al., "Adverse Drug Events in Hospitalized Patients. Excess Length of Stay, Extra Costs, and Attributable Mortality," *JAMA,* 277, 1997, pp. 301–306.

[9]D. W. Bates et al., "Incidence of Adverse Drug Events and Potential Adverse Drug Events: Implications for Prevention," *JAMA,* 274(1), July 5, 1995, pp. 29–34.

Consider the following fictional example of a medication error. Dr. Jones writes an antibiotic order to treat a possible pneumonia at 10:30 p.m. for a patient that reads, "Ampicillin 250 mg every 8 hours, give the first dose stat." The physician does not inform the nursing staff that the order has been written. The nurse finally notices the drug order at 4 a.m. Since she is alarmed that the order has been ignored for so long, she takes the order directly to the pharmacy. The pharmacy computer system is "down" for the usual nightly maintenance, so the pharmacist is unable to check to see if the patient has allergies to the medication. The nurse assures the pharmacist that the patient has no allergies. The pharmacist agrees to dispense two 250-mg ampicillin capsules.

WHAT ARE THE POTENTIAL MEDICATION ERRORS?

- Was this the right drug? *Although the correct drug was dispensed, the nurse determined, upon questioning the patient, that he had an allergy to penicillin. In addition, it would have been determined, had the appropriate lab reports been reviewed, that the offending bacterium was not susceptible to this antibiotic.*
- Was this the right dose? *Had this been the correct drug, the dose would have been inadequate to treat the intended indication.*
- Was this the right route? *The physician intended the drug to be administered intravenously but omitted the route from the order. Appropriate procedure would require that unclear orders be verified with the prescribing physician. The oral route was incorrectly implied by the pharmacist and is an inappropriate route to treat the intended indication.*
- Was this the right patient? *This is the only aspect of this medication order that was correct.*
- Was the drug administered at the right time? *A significant and inappropriate delay occurred in the administration of the drug. A $5\frac{1}{2}$-hour delay in drug administration could be life threatening in some situations.*

Although this example is a bit contrived, it illustrates the process and the potential for errors in drug administration. It is clear that important information can be derived from drug administration and pharmacy records to confirm the presence of a medication error.

THE MEDICATION DISTRIBUTION PROCESS

The following are general steps involved in the medication distribution process for a new medication order:

- Physician or provider generates a medication order
- Nursing staff acts on the order
- Order is sent to pharmacy department
- Pharmacist reviews order and dispenses medication
- Medication arrives in the patient-care area
- Medication is administered to the patient

PHYSICIAN OR PROVIDER GENERATES MEDICATION ORDER

In one study of preventable medication errors in adults, 56% occurred at ordering, 34% at administration, 6% at transcribing, and 4% at dispensing.[10] Since more than half of medication errors begin in the ordering stage and physician orders are well documented, the physician order sheet should be a major focus of the medical chart reviewer.

When a prescriber writes an order for a medication, it initiates a complex chain of events involving multiple departments and multiple professionals. These events are documented in both temporary and permanent records. Professionals who have been given prescriptive authority by the state may write medication orders. The professionals who are typically authorized to write prescriptions include physicians (interns and residents), physician assistants, nurse practitioners, nurses, pharmacists, optometrists, and podiatrists.

NURSING STAFF ACTS ON THE ORDER

Once the physician writes an order, the nursing staff manually transcribes it into a medication administration record (MAR). This step is omitted when computerized prescriber order entry (CPOE) is used. Then the nurse forwards the order to the pharmacy for review and dispensing. The nurse has a responsibility to review medication orders for obvious contraindications, dosage errors, or patient allergies before forwarding the order to the pharmacy.

Certain medications may be administered directly from a secured location on the nursing unit. These medications may be stored in a locked medication cabinet or available from an automated dispensing system (ADS). The retrieval of medications from a locked cabinet is not routinely documented unless the drug to be administered is a controlled substance. By contrast, any medication retrieved from an automated dispensing system unit will generate a record of removal.

---

[10]D. W. Bates et al., "Incidence of Adverse Drug Events and Potential Adverse Drug Events: Implications for Prevention," *JAMA,* 274(1), July 5, 1995, pp. 29–34.

Automated Dispensing Systems

Examples of ADSs include PYXIS and Omnicell. ADSs work like ATMs. They open a drawer or "pocket" filled with a specific medication when a particular patient and medication is selected. ADSs may be stand-alone systems or integrated with the electronic pharmacy system. Stand-alone systems allow removal of medications without review by a pharmacist. Integrated systems require a pharmacist to verify the order before the drug is "released" to be dispensed to the patient. The type of system used by a given institution may vary. An emergency department may have a stand-alone system, but access to controlled substances on nursing units may require verification. This verification process can be overridden, especially if 24-hour pharmacy services are not available. A log of over- rides is generated daily and reviewed by a pharmacist. Dispensing records are also generated from the ADS units, although those records are not part of the permanent medical record. ADS records are maintained by the pharmacy department in either paper or electronic form. The duration of storage of the records can vary. Controlled-substance records must be maintained for a minimum of two years. The following informa- tion is contained in ADS reports:

- Patient name and identification number
- Identity of the individual removing the medication
- Name and strength of the medication removed
- Time the medication is removed
- Physician name (may not always be the actual ordering physician, but rather the admitting physician)

An ADS facilitates medication distribution and reduces drug diversion. These systems do not, however, eliminate the potential for medication errors. The following are typical errors that may occur when using an ADS:

- Incorrect medication placed in the ADS.
- Incorrect medication removed from system. *This would be more likely to occur in a system that does not require pharmacist verification or when the override option is used.*
- Patient has an allergy to the medication administered. *This would be more likely to occur in a system that does not require pharmacist verifi- cation or when an override is used.*
- Incorrect patient receives the medication.

PHARMACIST REVIEWS ORDER AND DISPENSES MEDICATION

Dispensing in Institutions without CPOE

Medication orders arrive in the pharmacy via scanner, fax, and automated or hand delivery. Most institutions have established methods to allow rapid delivery. Copies of orders that arrive in the pharmacy may be saved for a limited period of time (i.e., 7–10 days). Orders with "problems" or those that require intervention may be saved for longer periods of time. Orders received in the pharmacy are not part of the permanent patient record. However, if a lawsuit is brought very soon after an accident, a request for this documentation can be made successfully.

Most pharmacies have a computer system that can access and update the patient's medication profile. The patient's *medication profile* is a list, created by the pharmacy, of all the medications that the patient has been prescribed during this hospitalization. These pharmacy systems may also interface with other computer databases to add lab and demographic data into the medication profile. Lab and demographic data are often important in the evaluation of the appropriateness of a medication order.

The addition of an order into the patient's electronic medication profile is usually the pharmacist's responsibility. However, some states may allow technicians to perform this task. Regardless of who physically enters the order into the computer, the pharmacist is ultimately responsible for ensuring the accuracy of the entry and the appropriateness of the order for a given patient. The computer record will indicate who entered and verified the order. With the addition of a new order in the medication profile, the pharmacist confirms that the drug is appropriate for the patient with regard to allergies, policy, dosage, and potential drug interactions. Most computer programs will prompt the pharmacist to review the aforementioned factors. Once the order is complete, two labels are generated, one for dispensing and one to be placed in the MAR.

Dispensing in Institutions with CPOE

Orders "arrive" in the pharmacy electronically via computer terminals located inside and outside of the hospital. With CPOE, the pharmacist no longer has to add the new drug to the patient's medication profile; the computer system does this automatically. The process of determining the appropriateness of the order occurs at both the physician and pharmacist level. The pharmacy order system provides electronic "prompts" to the ordering physician. These prompts suggest appropriate dosages and warn about contraindications and possible drug-drug interactions, etc. The pharmacist will have similar prompts on his terminal, helping to verify the appropriateness of the drug before he or she dispenses it. An exception to this review process occurs when "immediate," "stat," or "one-time" orders are made.

Medication Dispensing

Medications are dispensed based on the computer-generated label and placed into bags for delivery to the nursing unit. Almost all oral medications are dispensed as "unit doses," with each tablet or capsule being packaged individually and labeled with the drug name, strength, manufacturer, lot number, and expiration date. Intravenous medications may be compounded in the pharmacy and are individually labeled. Delivery to the nursing units occurs at scheduled intervals. Medications requiring more immediate patient administration may be available in a secure area on the nursing unit.

MEDICATION ARRIVES IN THE PATIENT-CARE AREA

The delivery of medication from the pharmacy to the nursing unit occurs at regularly scheduled intervals. A pharmacy technician or courier usually completes the delivery. Since the delivery schedule is predetermined, nursing staff will not be routinely notified that medication has arrived. All medications include a label identifying the patient's name. Documentation of this part of the medication distribution process would be minimal and is not part of the permanent patient record.

MEDICATION IS ADMINISTERED TO THE PATIENT

As part of the redundant review system, the nurse shares the responsibility to ensure that the drug delivered to the patient is correct. The nurse compares the MAR label that was generated in the pharmacy to the medication order and also compares the medication received to the original order. This verification is recorded in the MAR. The verification is signaled by the nurse initialing the newly arrived MAR label. However, the process may vary from institution to institution. Once the nurse is satisfied the correct medication has arrived, it should be administered to the patient at the next closest dosage time. In order to ensure appropriate dosing intervals, most medications are administered in accord with a standardized schedule on the hospital floor. These standard administration times will appear in a specific policy and may include unique administration times for particular drugs. Standard administration times are recorded in military time, to prevent confusion between a.m. and p.m. doses. In cases where a medication error is suspected, the reviewer should request a copy of the facility's drug administration policies for review and comparison against events recorded in the chart.

The following is an example of a list of standard administration times:

Interval	Time
QD (daily)	0800
BID (twice daily)	0800, 2000
TID (three times daily)	0800, 1400, 2000
Q 8h (every 8 hours)	0800, 1600, 2400

MEDICATION IS ADMINISTERED TO THE PATIENT

As noted previously, more than one-third of medication errors occur at the time of administration. Many people can administer medication in the hospital setting (e.g., physicians, residents, medical students, or patients). However, the nursing staff handle the majority of drug administration tasks.

Medications may be administered by various routes. (See Table 25.1.) It is also the responsibility of the nurse to ensure the administration occurs according to policy. Nurses traditionally are trained in subcutaneous, intramuscular, and intravenous routes of drug administration. Certain routes of drug administration are handled exclusively by physicians; for example, intracardiac, intrathecal, or intraocular routes. Nurses document their drug administrations in the MAR. Physicians document their drug administrations in progress or procedure notes.

Documentation of Medication Orders and Administration

The following are examples and explanations of documents that are used by physicians, nurses, and pharmacists in the clinical setting.

Medication Orders

To be correctly filled, a drug order must have the following information:

- Time (when the order is written)
- Date (when the order is written)
- Name of drug (chemical name or brand name)
- Dose (number of milligrams or cubic centimeters of drug in each administration)
- Frequency and/or timing of administrations (one single dose, twice a day, three times per day, after meals, at time of sleep, etc.)
- Route of administration (orally, intravenously, intramuscularly, etc.)
- Signature of prescriber

Table 25.1   Routes of Administration

Term	Site
Oral	Mouth (implies swallowing)
Sublingual	Under the tongue
Buccal	Oral cavity (between cheek and gums)
Enteral Tubes (Multiple types of tubes exist including nasogastric, nasoduodenal, nasojejunal, gastric, or jejunal)	GI tract
Topical (epicutaneous)	Skin surface
Intraocular, conjunctival	Eye
Intranasal	Nose
Aural	Ear
Inhalation, intrarespiratory	Lung
Rectal	Rectum
Intravaginal	Vagina
Intraurethral	Urethral
Parenteral Routes	
Intravenous	Vein
Intraarterial	Artery
Intramuscular	Muscle
Subcutaneous	Beneath the skin
Intradermal	Skin (dermis)
Intraspinal, intrathecal, epidural	Spine
Intracardiac	Heart
Intraosseous	Bone
Intraarticular	Joint
Intrasynovial	Joint-fluid area

The order-writing process is dependent on the type of medical record used by the institution. An order may be generated either in the traditional written form or through a CPOE.

Medication Administration Records

The MAR is a document that contains the names of medications that were administered to a given patient at a specified time. This document is created by the nursing staff to remind them which medications the patient is currently taking and which medications must be administered. Each patient has a unique MAR. The individual administering the medication will initial or sign the MAR to indicate the dose was administered. All initials should be clarified with a signature sheet. A medication is not considered administered if it is not recorded on the MAR.

Several different types of MARs may exist. (See Table 25.2.) Certain MARs are generated from the electronic pharmacy record. The frequency at which the MARs are generated differs depending on the institution and the patient-care unit. The frequency can vary from daily to every 30 days. This process serves as a reconciliation between the nursing and pharmacy medication transcriptions. Newly generated MARs must be reviewed by the nurse, and any discrepancies must be reported to the

Table 25.2   Medication Administration Records

MAR Type	Type of Documentation
Standard	Routine, recurring orders
PRN	Medication ordered as needed, most often for pain and nausea/vomiting.
One-time orders	Medication ordered for one time or single dose administration. Includes immediate or "stat" orders
Procedural	Medication administered during diagnostic or invasive procedures such as surgery, angiography, endoscopy, and others
Flow sheets	Medication administered through a continuous intravenous solution
Medication specific	Medication requiring nursing driven dose adjustment based on specific parameters such as anticoagulants and insulins
Code sheets	Medication administered during a cardiac arrest or other acute life-threatening event requiring mobilization of an advanced life support team
Electronic	All medication administered verified with Bar coding. See text.

pharmacy. When reviewing the MARs, it is important to note the point at which the new MARs arrive in the patient chart and if any errors were reported. The MAR and signature sheet are part of the patient's permanent medical record.

Traditional Charting System

Orders generated in a traditional system are handwritten on preprinted order sheets. Handwritten orders are subject to many errors, including those that arise from illegible writing, incomplete knowledge of the prescriber, and lapses in the prescriber's judgment. The medication order must be transcribed by the nurse and, subsequently, the pharmacist prior to drug administration. This transcription allows two more opportunities for transcription errors. The careful chart reviewer will compare the drug order written in the physician order sheet with that written by the nurse and the pharmacist.

Once the physician writes the order, he or she is obligated to notify the nursing staff that a new order has been placed on the chart. This is especially true if the new order requires immediate administration (i.e., a "stat" order). Although the physician may write "stat" on the medication order sheet, his contemporaneous verbal notification is not routinely documented. A flag or other physical indicator (usually found in the outside area of the chart) is sufficient notification for routine orders.

Computerized Physician Order Entry Systems

CPOE eliminates many of the problems associated with traditional medication order systems. CPOE provides information on appropriate prescribing indications, dosing, allergies, and potential drug interactions, and reduces the time for order processing. Computerized orders are, generally, printed and placed in the chart for reference. Most orders are reviewed and verified by a pharmacist prior to dispensing, but some exceptions exist.

Computerized order entry systems have the ability to recognize inappropriate dosages of medication, drug-drug interactions, drug-pregnancy interactions, and drug allergies. These CPOE systems are designed to prevent the entry of prescriptions that may be dangerous to the patient. However, prescribers may override electronic warnings when the clinical situation dictates. These overrides are stored in the computer system and are available for review later. If a medication error is suspected as a cause of patient injury, the pharmacy system override log should be requested and reviewed. Storage and retention of electronic records must comply with state laws governing the permanent medical record.

Electronic Pharmacy Records (Institutions without CPOE)

The duration of storage of the electronic pharmacy record may differ from institution to institution. Most records will be available for at least one year. These records are not part of the permanent patient record. The pharmacy record will generate MARs (see below) that become a part of the permanent record.

What to Evaluate in the Electronic Pharmacy Records

* Time from written order to pharmacy order entry
* Compare written (non-CPOE) and electronic orders
* Drug interactions (flagged during electronic order entry)
* Dosage recommendations (flagged during electronic order entry)
* ADS records

Paper Pharmacy Records

Most pharmacy departments *will not keep* patient-specific paper records for extended periods. Written information that applies to a specific patient will be discarded after a patient is discharged. This written information often includes forms the pharmacist uses to track patient response to drug therapy.

Pharmacy departments that use an entirely manual system to dispense medication and generate MARs are unusual. In the event the pharmacy does not use an electronic medication profile, all orders are transcribed by hand. Again, these records are not maintained after patient discharge. After a specified period of time of hospitalization (i.e., one week), manual profiles maintained by the pharmacy may generate a MAR. In these instances, the pharmacy would type the manual MAR and provide a copy for the permanent record.

The pharmacy department uses a minimal amount of paper records. Those records that are used are destroyed soon after the patient is discharged. The pharmacy may, however, retain these records for an unspecified period of time for quality assurance or data collection. It is important for the chart reviewer to determine what paper records are routinely saved and whether or not they are still available for review.

Each department will develop and utilize forms to meet its specific needs; therefore a complete list of standardized documents is not possible. The following are examples of frequently used paper forms.

Non-formulary medication orders

These are used to help track the request and procurement of non-formulary medications. A *non-formulary item* is one that the institution does not routinely stock, and it usually requires a special request from the ordering physician. A copy of the hospital's formulary should be available for review in the pharmacy department or on any nursing unit.

Special medication profiles

If a medication or therapeutic regimen requires special compounding and/or monitoring, the pharmacy may use an alternate medication profile to track dispensing and monitor response to therapy. The profile may contain a copy of the pharmacy order, lab values, and other parameters pertinent to the medication being dispensed. Policies may also exist that discuss the use of these profiles and/or the pharmacist's response to given parameters. Common medications that may have a special profile include anticoagulants, chemotherapeutic agents, and parenteral nutrition solutions. Special medication profiles are often discarded after a patient has been discharged. Sometimes these records are retained for quality-assurance purposes and may be discoverable.

"Problem orders"

Pharmacy departments routinely track the number of orders that must be clarified prior to dispensing the medication. These orders may be referred to as "problem orders," or interventions. Some departments may keep problem orders in a paper format, while others might develop a database tracking program. If the latter is used, patient identifiers may be removed from the database. In either event, the process by which problem orders are identified and documented should be discovered to determine if an enduring record exists.

Controlled substance administration records

Paper records are generated in hospitals that do not use ADS and when controlled substances are administered as continuous infusions.

Documentation of Medication Errors

If a medication error is noted immediately, it may be recorded in several places, including a pharmacy "medication error report," an "adverse drug event report," and a "nursing incident report."

Incident report

This report describes the incident, the people involved, and the circumstances. The incident report is created by the nursing department for quality-assurance purposes, but may be discoverable (see Chapter 24).

Medication error report

The pharmacy should also record all medication errors. A medication error report should contain information about the drug, dose, timing, people involved, nature of error, and circumstances surrounding the error. The medication error report is stored in the pharmacy, and it may be available for discovery. (See Figure 25.1.)

Adverse drug event report

This is a report of all adverse drug events that the pharmacy department is made aware of. It is important to emphasize the difference between a medication error report and an adverse drug event report. *Adverse drug events* are those events where an appropriate medication administration (i.e., the correct drug, dose, route, patient, etc.) resulted in patient injury, such as allergic reaction, liver function abnormalities, arrhythmias, etc. Adverse drug reaction reports do not focus on possible negligence committed by physicians or nurses, but, rather, on the patient's reactions to medication. Adverse reactions to medications are reportable to the drug manufacturer and the Food and Drug Administration.

High-Risk Medications

Published studies of adverse drug events and multiple case reports have consistently identified certain classes of medications as particularly serious threats to patient safety.[11,12,13] These high-risk medications include concentrated electrolyte solutions (such as potassium chloride), intravenous insulin, chemotherapeutic agents, intravenous opiate analgesics, and anticoagulants (such as heparin and warfarin). Analyses of some of the adverse events involving these medications have led to important recommendations for improving safety in their administration. The hospital is expected to exercise special care with regard to storage, preparation, label-

[11]D. W. Bates et al., "Incidence of Adverse Drug Events and Potential Adverse Drug Events: Implications for Prevention," *JAMA,* 274(1), July 5, 1995, pp. 29–34.

[12]M. R. Cohen et al., "Preventing Medication Errors in Cancer Chemotherapy," *Am J Health Syst Pharm,* 53, 1996, pp. 737–746.

[13]T. A. Brennan et al., "Incidence of Adverse Events and Negligence in Hospitalized Patients. Results of the Harvard Medical Practice Study I," *N Engl J Med,* 324, 1991, pp. 370–376.

Acme Hospital

Medication Error Report

☐ Not Part of the Medical Record
☐ For Quality Assurance Purposes Only

Patient Name: _____

Ward: _____

Date:_____

Date of Report _____

Date/Time of Notification _____

Reporting individual: (Cirlce one. Do not include names)
RN   RP   MD   Other _____

☐ Nurse Manager   ☐ Shift Nursing Supervisor
☐ Pharmacist   ☐ Physician

Type of Event (Check all that apply) Date/Time of Error: _____

Ordering:

___A. Inappropriate med(s)	___E. Order not dated/timed
___B. Inappropriate dose	___F. Wrong chart
___C. Illegible	___G. Contraindication (e.g. allergy)
___D. Duplication	___H. Verbal order misunderstood

___I. Verbal order not in chart
___J. Non-formulary
___K. Other (explain on back)

Transcription Error:

___A. Wrong medication	___E. Wrong duration
___B. Wrong time	___F. Wrong patient
___C. Wrong dose	___G. Wrong chart
___D. Wrong frequency	___H. Verbal order misunderstood

___I. Verbal order not in chart
___J. Other (explain on back)
___K. Order not on MAR

Preparation/Dispensing:

___A. Inaccurate labeling	___E. Wrong dose
___B. Wrong quantity	___F. Delay in delivery
___C. Wrong medication	___G. Wrong time

___I. Wrong frequency
___J. Other (explain on back)

Administration:

___A. Wrong patient	___E. Wrong medication
___B. Wrong dose	___F. Omission
___C. Wrong time	___G. Commission

___I. Other (explain on back)

Severity of Event: (must choose one category)

✔	Type of Error/Category	Result
	No Error	
	Category A	Circumstances or events that have the capacity to cause error.
	Error, No Harm	
	Category B	An error occurred but the medication did not reach the patient
	ITEMS BELOW REQUIRE IMMEDIATE ACTION	
	**Category C	An error occurred that reached the patient but did not cause patient harm.
	**Category D	An error occurred that resulted in the need for increased monitoring but no patient harm.
	Error, Harm	
	**Category E	An error occurred that resulted in the need for treatment or intervention and caused temporary patient harm.
	**Category F	An error occurred that resulted in initial or prolonged hospitalization and caused patient harm.
	**Category G	An error occurred that resulted in permanent patient harm.
	**Category H	An error occurred that resulted in near-death event (e.g., anaphylaxis, cardiac arrest)
	Error, Death	
	**Category I	An error occurred that resulted in patient death.

**Physician findings and orders (For Category C through Category I). _____

Signature _____ M.D.

Forward before end of shift:

Nurse Manager:	Time/Date _____	Signature _____
Director of Nursing:	Time/Date _____	Signature _____
Pharmacy:	Time/Date _____	Signature _____
Risk Manager:	Time/Date _____	Signature _____

Figure 25.1   Example of Medication Error Report

ing, dispensation, and administration of these medications. This special care is usually formalized as hospital policy. Policies relating to administration of medication, especially high-alert medications, would not be part of the patient's medical record. In cases of medical injury where a medication error is suspected, the medical chart reviewer should review the physician's order sheet and MAR for any of these high-risk medications. A copy of the hospital and pharmacy policies on the use and administration of these drugs should be requested. The reviewer should compare the policies on these issues against actual events in the case under review.

Medications that are frequently involved in medication errors are in the Institute of Safe Medical Practices' list of high-alert medications. (See Table 25.3.) High-alert medications have received this designation due to repeated reports of errors of inappropriate administration and the resultant patient injuries.

WHAT ARE THE DIFFERENT TYPES OF MEDICATION ORDERS?

Medications may be ordered for immediate, one-time, recurring, or as-needed administration. The type of order may determine the distribution and administration process.

Table 25.3   High-Alert or High-Risk Medications

Category and Route of Administration	Example
Adrenergic agonists, intravenous	epinephrine, dopamine
Adrenergic antagonists, intravenous	propranolol, metoprolol, esmolol
Anesthetic agents, inhaled and intravenous	propofol, halothane
Cardioplegic agents, intravenous	electrolyte containing solutions used for cardiac bypass surgery
Chemotherapeutic Agents, oral and parenteral	methotrexate, vincristine, cisplatin
Dextrose, hypertonic 20% or greater	parenteral solutions used to compound intravenous nutrition solutions
Dialysis solutions, hemodialysis and peritoneal	nonphysiologic electrolyte solutions
Epidural or intrathecal medications	pain medications, antibiotics, chemotherapeutic agents
Glycoprotein IIb/IIIa inhibitors, intravenous	eptifibatide, abciximab, tirofiban
Hypoglycemics, oral, subcutaneous, intravenous	glipizide, glyburide, insulin
Inotropic medication, intravenous	digoxin, dobutamine, milrinone

Liposomal dosage forms, intravenous	liposomal amphotericin B
Moderate sedation agents, intravenous	lorazepam, midazolam
Moderate sedation agents, oral, children	chloral hydrate
Narcotics and opiates, oral and intravenous	codeine, morphine, meperidine
Neuromuscular blocking agents	atracurium, succinylcholine, vecuronium
Radiocontrast agents, intravenous	
Thrombolytics/fibrinolytics, intravenous	alteplase, reteplase, streptokinase, tenecteplase
Total parenteral nutrition solutions	intravenous solutions containing electrolytes, protein, glucose +/− fat
Specific Medications	**Indication /Use**
Amiodarone, intravenous	anti-arrhythmic
Colchicine injection	acute gout
Heparin, intravenous	anticoagulant
Heparin, low-molecular weight, injection	anticoagulant
Insulin, subcutaneous, intravenous	diabetes, high blood glucose
Lidocaine, intravenous	anti-arrhythmic
Magnesium sulfate injection	anti-arrhythmic, electrolyte replacement, preterm labor
Nesiritide	acute heart failure
Nitroprusside sodium injection	acute heart failure, hypertension
Potassium chloride injection, concentrated	electrolyte replacement
Potassium phosphates injection	electrolyte replacement
Sodium chloride injection, hypertonic, concentration more than 0.9%	correction of hyponatremia, volume expansion
Sterile water for injection, large volume parenteral	used for compounding only, never for direct administration to patients
Warfarin	anticoagulant

The list of examples is not intended to be all inclusive. Please consult a drug reference source to obtain a complete list.

Source: Adapted from the Institute for Safe Medication Practices Website. URL http://www.ismp.org/MSAarticles/HighAlertPrint.htm.

Immediate Orders

Immediate, or "stat," orders should be administered to patients within a prespecified time period. In general, institutions have policies dictating the window of administration, such as "within 30 minutes of the medication order." The majority of the time a "stat" medication order implies the need to address an urgent patient problem. Medications in this category may be stored under controlled conditions on a nursing unit or require dispensing from the pharmacy.

Single Dose Orders

Single dose orders are intended for one time only. These orders are dispensed using the process previously described.

Recurring Orders

Recurring orders include regularly scheduled and as-needed orders. Initial orders are transcribed and dispensed as previously described. Subsequent medications are provided to patient-care areas in medication carts. Errors that occur during this part of the dispensing process are generally not documented in the patient record.

Orders for Controlled Substances

Orders for controlled substances, such as narcotic analgesics, are considered separately because all institutions have specific policies regarding the accounting and dispensing of these medications. The fate of each dose must be accounted for; thus a duplicate record of patient administration will be generated. Federal law requires that records are maintained for a minimum of two years, and state laws may have stricter requirements. Therefore, documentation of controlled substance administration can be found on both the patient's MAR and in controlled substance records. As controlled substances are also high-alert medications, the chart reviewer should request hospital and pharmacy policies on the handling and administration of these medications. Be alert to any policy on monitoring of patients after they've been medicated, as lack of monitoring after use of narcotics and sedatives can result in missing respiratory depression, a common cause of morbidity and mortality in these patients.

CONCLUSIONS

The medication distribution process is a complex system designed to minimize errors and, ultimately, patient harm. The process is not foolproof, and the potential for errors continues to exist despite safeguards. Several different types of records, both permanent and temporary, exist that can help identify whether an error has been made. For a list of documents the medical chart reviewer should request and review in a medication error case, see Table 25.4.

Table 25.4   Documents to Request on Cases of Suspected Medication Error

---

The following documents should be requested and reviewed when a case of negligent drug administration is suspected:

❑ Full medical chart including physician order sheets

❑ Medication administration report (MAR)

❑ Patient's medication profile

❑ "Special" medication profiles

❑ Pharmacy dispensing records (handwritten or electronic)

❑ Controlled substances administration record

❑ Hospital policies on drug orders, drug administration, medication error notifications and reports, and adverse drug reaction reports

❑ Pharmacy department policies on drug orders, drug administration, medication error reporting, and adverse drug reaction reporting

❑ Medication error reports

❑ Adverse drug reaction reports

❑ "Problem" medication orders (orders that require clarification from prescriber)

❑ Nursing incident report of administration errors

❑ Pharmacy ordering system override logs

❑ Non-formulary or "special" medication request logs

CHAPTER 26

The Medical Chart
as Evidence

This chapter will help explain the nature of the medical record as evidence and how this evidence is used in a court of law.

Q **What is evidence?**

A *Evidence* is the means by which an alleged matter of fact is established or disproved.

Q **How is the medical record used in a lawsuit?**

A A patient's medical records are very often crucial evidence in a variety of settings in a lawsuit. For example, the medical record can be used to provide the following information:

- Injury causation in a personal injury suit
- The extent of damages in a personal injury suit
- The due care, or lack of due care, in a medical malpractice suit
- Relevant information about a patient's condition[1]
- That the patient gave informed consent, or, conversely, suggest that the patient did not give informed consent

---

[1]For example, a patient was intoxicated in the case of *Campbell v. Manhattan and Bronx Transit Operating Authority,* 812 A.D.2d 529, 438 N.Y.S. 2d 87 (1st Dept 1981), and this condition of intoxication was pertinent along with diagnosis and treatment.

Q   **What is hearsay?**

A   *Hearsay* is a type of testimony given by a witness who relates, not to what he or she knows personally, but to what others have told him or her, or what he or she heard said by others. In such cases, that knowledge is dependent on the credibility of the other person, who cannot be examined in court, and, as such, it is not admissible in court unless it meets the criteria for an exception to the hearsay rule.

Q   **What is the "hearsay rule?"**

A   The *hearsay rule* is a rule of evidence that generally prohibits a person from providing testimony based upon what that person has been told or learned secondhand. The rules of evidence favor testimony based upon a person's own observations.

Q   **How are medical charts admitted as evidence in a trial?**

A   As a general proposition, medical records are considered hearsay; that is, statements contained in the records are, in effect, "out-of-court" declarations. For medical records to be admitted into evidence at trial, legal counsel must lay an adequate foundation, which may include an exception to the hearsay rule.

Q   **What does the term "laying a foundation" mean?**

A   *"Laying a foundation"* for evidence refers to introducing preliminary proof to establish that evidence is admissible. Laying a foundation for the admissibility of a medical record, or any document, consists of demonstrating what the record is and how it was made. Only after a document is admitted into evidence may a witness talk about what the document actually says.

Q   **Does a witness always have to testify to lay the foundation for a medical record?**

A   No. It is always proper (and often a good idea), for the physician or other medical professional who wrote the record to lay the foundation by taking the witness stand. However, if the author physician is not available, a records custodian or office manager, under some circumstances, may present an adequate foundation through live testimony. In other instances, records properly certified by the producing entity may be admitted into evidence without any live testimony.

Q   **What are the different types of medical records recognized by the courts?**

A   The decision by the Appellate Division, Second Department, in *Wilson v. Bodian*,[2] recognized and drew distinctions between three basic types of medical records: hospital records, physician's records, and physician's reports that are prepared for the case.

Q   **Are hospital records admissible evidence in court?**

A   Hospital records are admissible without a foundation witness, if copies produced by the hospital bear a certification or authentication by the head of the hospital, an employee delegated for that purpose, or a qualified physician. According to Civil Practice Law and Rules (CPLR) 4518(c), a statutory exception to the hearsay rule, hospital records are *prima facie* evidence of the facts contained in them, once admitted.

Q   **Are physician's office records admissible as evidence?**

A   Records kept by a physician in the course of diagnosis and treatment of a patient are business records. Business records may be admitted into evidence pursuant to CPLR 4518 (a), another statutory exception to the hearsay rule. If the physician's records are certified in accordance with CPLR 3122-a (a), then the records may be admitted into evidence without testimony from the physician or any other live witness. CPLR 3122-a (a) prescribes[3] the affidavit required for the records to be admitted into evidence. In substance, CPLR 3122-a (a) requires the following to be true:

- The affiant is the duly authorized custodian or other-qualified witness and has authority to make the certification.
- To the best of the affiant's knowledge, the records, after a reasonable inquiry, are accurate copies of the subpoenaed documents in the custodian's possession.

---

[2] *Wilson v. Bodian*, 130 A.D.2d 221, 229, 519 N.Y.S.2d 126, 131 (2nd Dep't 1987).

[3] The affidavit required by CPLR 3122-1 (a) is quite specific, in contrast to the fairly general language of CPLR 4581 (c), which merely requires "certification or authentication."

- To the best of the affiant's knowledge, the records produced, after reasonable inquiry, are all the records called for in the subpoena, or absences are adequately explained.
- The records were made by personnel, staff, or persons under their control in the regular course of business, and the records were made at the time of the act or event was recorded or within a reasonable time thereafter.

CPLR 3122(c) provides that the party offering the records without a witness must give notice of intent not later than 30 days before trial, and any party wishing to object to the records' admission must assert the objection and grounds not later than ten days before trial. Regardless of whether or not an objection was made, a party may subpoena the custodian of records to appear at trial with the original records. Legal counsel must make a tactical decision whether to use a live witness or go with certified copies of a medical record. A live witness is usually more interesting, and the medical professional who made the notes may offer additional testimony, if necessary.[4] On the other hand, using certified records simplifies counsel's life considerably by reducing problems with scheduling witnesses and curtailing expenses.

Q   **Are physician reports that are prepared for litigation admissible as evidence?**

A   Physician's reports prepared for litigation are inadmissible as evidence under the business records exception to the hearsay rule.[5] This is only logical, since the report was not prepared in the "ordinary course of business," but rather was prepared at the request of a lawyer.

It is important to note that the New York Uniform Rules of Court (22 NYCRR) section 202.17 provides for medical examination of claimants and exchange of medical reports by the physicians performing these examinations. Failure to comply can result in the preclusion of testimony by the examining physician. If a physician retained by a party wrote a report that was not terribly helpful to that party, the opposing counsel would love to use this report. However, since the report itself is hearsay (i.e., not within

---

[4]For example, see discussion of *Wilson v. Bodian*, infra.
[5]*Wilson v. Bodian*, 130 A.D.2d 221, 229, 519 N.Y.S.2d 126, 131 (2nd Dep't 1987).

the "business records exception"), it cannot be put into evidence. If the party who retained the examining physician does not put him or her on the stand to testify, opposing counsel could subpoena the physician to testify. Once the physician is on the stand, counsel can confront the physician with his or her report and offer the findings in the report into evidence.

Q   **Why is an expert witness called to testify in court about medical care?**

A   Even if certified medical records are allowed into evidence without a live witness, it may still be necessary to call a witness to explain them. In fact, not calling a live witness to adequately interpret the records may result in reversal. For example, in *Wilson v. Bodian* (a medical malpractice case), the records of a physician who had examined the plaintiff (patient) before she was seen by the defendant (physician) had been offered and admitted into evidence. One particularly important issue was whether the defendant physician had known that a biopsy had been previously performed on the patient. The admitted records contained the notation "BX," which the patient's counsel argued meant that a biopsy had indeed been performed and that the defendant physician, who had read the records, should have know this. However, neither the defendant physician nor his expert acknowledged that "BX" was a commonly understood abbreviation for biopsy. The patient's counsel told the court that the physician who had written the notation had not responded to a subpoena to testify at trial, but the patient's counsel did not have the process server testify and did not offer an affidavit of service to establish that the physician had been properly subpoenaed. The custodian witness that laid the foundation for the records authenticity was not a medical person and did not know what the notation meant. The appellate court found, "[u]nlike hospital records which contain generally accepted and standard medical abbreviations, a physician's office records may contain purely personal abbreviations known only to the physician."[6] The court held that to allow into evidence the "BX" notation, "which abbreviation is not within the ken of the jury, in the absence of the physician author, there must be a foundation laid

---

[6]*Wilson* at 232, 519 N.Y.S.2d at 133.

that such an abbreviation has a well-known and accepted meaning in the medical profession. An abbreviation of this kind that is not interpretable as having a definite and accepted meaning is not admissible."[7] Thus, even though the physician's office records as a whole were admissible as business records, the "BX" notation was improper before the jury. The problem was aggravated when the patient's counsel argued in summation that "BX" meant biopsy. Ultimately, the appellate court reversed a verdict for the patient and ordered a new trial.

Q **Are there any other types of information in the medical record that are not admissible as evidence?**

A Information noted in the medical record that is not necessary for the patient's diagnosis, prognosis, treatment, or otherwise helpful to an understanding of the medical or surgical aspects of a patient's hospitalization, such as detailed narratives of how an accident happened related by the patient, is not necessarily within the hearsay exception.[8] For example, a patient's statement in a narrative that a car hit him or her may be admissible under the hearsay exception, but the statement that he or she was hit within the crosswalk and that the car went through a red light would not be admissible.

Q **How are illegible or unreadable notes handled in a lawsuit?**

A Unfortunately, portions of medical records are not always legible. If this is so, the illegible portions should be redacted to avoid confusing the jury. However, relevant legible parts of a record need not necessarily be excluded merely because other parts are illegible. In *Campbell v. Manhattan and Bronx Transit Operation Authority*,[9] the appellate court held that the trial court improperly excluded a legible portion of a hospital record dealing with a patient's inability to give a history due to intoxication and ordered a new trial.

---

[7]*Id.* at 232, 519 N.Y.S.2d at 133.

[8]*Wilson v. Alexander*, 309 N.Y. 283, 287, 129 N.E.2d 417, 419 (1955).

[9]*Campbell v. Manhattan and Bronx Transit Operation Authority*, 81 A.D.2d 329, 438 N.Y.S. 2d 87 (1st Dep't 1981).

Q   **Are graphic materials, such as radiographs, MRIs, photographs, and drawings, admissible as evidence?**

A   CPLR 4532-a provides that "graphic, numerical, symbolic or pictorial representations of medical or diagnostic tests in personal injury actions" are admissible as exceptions to the hearsay rule, as long as they have the following information inscribed on them:

- Patient's name
- Date taken
- Identifying number
- Name and address of supervising physician

This provision applies to X-rays, MRIs, CT scans, positron emission tomography (PET) scans, electromyograms (EMGs), sonograms, fetal heart monitor recordings, as well as anything else that medical science has been able to dream up that fits the statute's description. The statute provides that if ten days' notice is given to the other side, along with an affidavit of the supervising physician, then the materials may be introduced into evidence without having to put the person who did the test on the witness stand.

If the materials do not have the proper inscription, they should not be allowed into evidence. In *Galuska v. Abaiza,*[10] the appellate court held that five X-rays that did not have the patient's name were improperly admitted and ordered a new trial on damages.

Q   **What is the best evidence rule?**

A   The *best evidence rule* requires that, for a document to be entered into evidence, it must be the original document, unless the original document is unavailable. If the unavailability of the original is adequately explained, copies or secondary evidence of what was in the original are sometimes allowed.

Q   **How does the best evidence rule apply to medical records?**

A   If the contents of a document are in dispute, the best evidence rule requires that the proponent produce the original document or offer an adequate explanation for why the original is not available. This rule extends to all manner of medical records includ-

---

[10]*Galuska v. Abaiza,* 106 A.D.2d 543, 482, 846 (2nd Dep't 1984).

ing graphic materials, such as X-rays. However, if there is a good explanation for why the original is not available, a copy or sometimes even a piece of secondary evidence may be used to show what was in the original. In *Schozer v. William Penn Life Insurance Co.,*[11] an original X-ray had been lost, and the lower courts excluded the X-ray report on the basis of the best evidence rule. However, the Court of Appeals, New York's highest court, held that this was an error and ordered a new trial. The Court of Appeals held that if the absence of the original, even an X-ray, was "excused, all competent secondary evidence is generally admissible to prove the original's contents ... provided its admission did not violate some other exclusionary rule or policy."[12] This opinion was not unanimous, the dissentors thought that allowing the X-ray report into evidence was improper since the report was not subject to cross-examination, and it put before the jury the expert opinion of the person who wrote the report. Nevertheless, this is currently the law in New York.

Q   **Can photocopies of medical documents be used as evidence in court?**

A   Notwithstanding the best evidence rule, photocopies of medical records may be used as evidence, rather than the originals, as long as all parties agree. This accommodation is routinely made in courts every day. If the parties cannot agree, however, the best evidence rule may apply. CPLR 4539, *Reproductions of Original,* provides that if any institution (such as a hospital) or member of a profession (such as a physician) kept records in the regular course of business and, in the regular course of business, copied those records by any process that accurately produced the original, then "such reproduction, when satisfactorily identified, is as admissible in evidence as the original, whether the original is in existence or not." The appellate court explains in *People v. May,*[13] that "CPLR 4539 carves out an exception to the best evidence rule for business records that are copied or reproduced, on the rationale that, in today's commercial world, the accuracy of such copies is relied on without question." This rule recog-

[11]*Schozer v. William Penn Life Insurance Co.*, 84 N.Y.2d 639, 620 N.Y.S.2d 797 (1994).
[12]*Id.* at 645, 620 N.Y.S.2d 800 (1994).
[13]*People v. May*, 162 A.D.2d 977, 977, 557, N.Y.S.2d 203, 204 (46th Dep't 1990).

nizes the fact that modern business practice is to make photographic reproductions during the regular course of business and that photographic reproductions so made are sufficiently trustworthy to be treated as originals for the purpose of the "best evidence rule."[14]

CPLR 2306(a) provides that where a *subpoena duces tecum* (i.e., a demand for documents usually issued by legal counsel for a party) is served on a hospital "requiring production of records relating to the condition or treatment of a patient, a transcript or full-sized legible reproduction certified as correct by the superintendent or head of the hospital ... or his assistant ... may be produced unless otherwise ordered by a court. Such a subpoena shall be served at least three days before the time fixed for the production of the records unless otherwise ordered by a court." As a practical matter, medical care providers are loathe to let original records out of their possession and invariably provide photocopies in response to *subpoenas deuces tecum*, unless the subpoena specified originals to be produced and the subpoena was signed "so ordered" by the court. If, after examining the photocopies, counsel believes it necessary to be able to look at the originals (e.g., if records are very light or otherwise not easily legible or there is a legitimate suspicion that the records were tampered with) counsel may obtain a court order requiring production of the originals.

Q   **Can electronic medical records be used as evidence in court?**

A   CPLR 4518(a), *Business Records*, provides that "an electronic record ... shall be admissible in a tangible exhibit that is a true and accurate representation of such electronic record. The court may consider the method or manner in which a record is stored, maintained, or retrieved in determining whether the exhibit is a true and accurate representation of such electronic record. All other circumstances of the making of the memorandum or record, including lack of personal knowledge by the maker, may be proved to affect its weight, but they shall not affect its admissibility." CPLR 4539(b) provides that "a reproduction created by

---

[14]*Id.* at 977, 557 N.Y.S.2d 204 (46th Dep't 1990).

any process which stores an image of any writing, entry, print, or representation and which does not permit additions, deletions, or changes without leaving a record of such additions, deletions, or changes, when authenticated by competent testimony or affidavit, which shall include the manner or method by which tampering or degradation of the reproduction is prevented, shall be as admissible in evidence as the original."

Thus, some medical records that are, by their nature, stored electronically (such as MRI optical discs), may be put into evidence by transferring the data onto a film and offering the film into evidence. This transfer may occur as long as an adequate foundation that the data have not been tampered with is laid.

CHAPTER 27

Tampering or Falsification?

INTRODUCTION

Most, both in and out of the medical community, believe that a physician has a duty to maintain the integrity, accuracy, truth, and reliability of the patient's medical record. They feel that the physician's obligation to the accuracy of the medical record is no less compelling than duties toward diagnosis and treatment of the patient, since other health care providers must, out of necessity, be able to rely on those records in the continuing and future care of that patient. It is with this in mind that legislators and the courts have held that a deliberate falsification by a physician of his or her patient's medical record is regarded as gross malpractice that endangers the health or life of the patient. This is particularly true when the reason for the change is to protect the physician's own interests at the expense of the patient's. In many states, the deliberate falsification of a medical record is criminal action.

Q **Who is responsible for the integrity of the medical chart?**

A The maintenance of medical charts is the responsibility of the author and the institution where the author works. The courts have held that there is a legal duty on the part of the hospital and its employees to exercise "reasonable care" in maintaining complete and accurate medical records. However, there is no consensus on how or how long these charts should be maintained.

What constitutes tampering with the medical record?

There exists a strong temptation, on the part of providers of medical care, to alter their entries in a chart when bad outcomes are observed or threats of legal liability become manifest.

Legally speaking, tampering with a medical record in a malpractice case constitutes a "spoliation of evidence." *Spoliation of evidence* is the failure to preserve property for another's use as evidence in a pending or future litigation. Spoliation may also include the alteration or fabrication of evidence to support one's cause, defense, or claim.

The following actions are considered acts of chart tampering:

- Removing records from the medical chart
- Adding fraudulent records to the medical chart
- Altering dates or facts in the medical chart
- Supplementing clinical notes at a later date, but using a contemporaneous date
- Altering or supplementing another health care provider's notes (e.g., physicians altering nurses' notes, and vice versa.)
- Purposely omitting significant clinical findings in the medical chart that would reflect badly on the provider of care
- Purposely adding fictitious clinical findings in the medical chart that would tend to support clinical reasoning or actions

Because of the easy access to the medical chart and speed that the hospital staff can detect a bad outcome, the medical chart is frequently altered. In fact, when discussing a notorious case of chart tampering, the U.S. Attorney Prosecutor David Hoffman admitted chart tampering to be a significant problem. He maintained that medical records are "routinely falsified" and that, if such falsifications were prosecuted as federal offenses, it would deter such behavior.[1]

What are the implications of chart tampering?

The term "spoliation of evidence" is derived from the Latin concept *omnia praesumuntur contra spoliatorem*, which means that all things are presumed against a suppressor of testimony. Therefore,

---

[1]R. Martin, "Falsification of Medical Records," *Advance for Nurses, Greater Philadelphia*, June 4, 2001, p. 44.

when a jury learns that the medical chart has been altered by the defendant, it implies that a mistake was made that needed to be hidden. This makes it difficult for the jury to see the defendant as anything but a guilty practitioner trying to hide his mistakes. Once the accuracy of the record is challenged, the integrity of the entire record becomes suspect. Malpractice cases are near impossible to win and settlements difficult to come by when chart tampering has been detected. The defense counsel may be required to settle the case out of court even if negligence hasn't occurred. When a plaintiff's attorney proves that chart tampering has taken place, the following outcomes may be possible:

- Extension of the statute of limitations based on the premise that fraud has been committed
- Imposition of court sanctions against defendants for failure to produce documents
- Punitive damages imposed if the defense counsel can argue that the medical chart was intentionally altered or lost because of conspiracy or fraud that constitutes "aggravated or outrageous conduct"

Q
A

How do you detect chart tampering?

The experienced chart reviewer will look for the following clues that may suggest chart tampering:

- Unnatural order of writing, uniformity of handwriting, changes in the color of the ink, use of margins, and change of word spacing.
- Intersecting fountain pen entries of different dates that bleed together.
- Differences between pages such as folds, stains, offsets, impressions, holes, tears, and type of paper used. *Medical charts are large objects that are moved about frequently and used by many personnel. These charts are subject to a variety of physical abuse in the hospital, office, and clinic. They absorb cuts, rips, burns, coffee, soda, and food stains. A pristine piece of paper in an otherwise well-used chart should be suspect.*
- Use of forms not available or commonly in use at the time of the purported entry.
- Use of a later year (such as 1999 for 1996), especially if it has been corrected several times.

- Medical records conflicting with the billing records. *Do bills appear for visits that are not recorded? Are visits recorded that have no bills associated with them?*
- Medication administration records conflicting with the nursing notes. *Do the nurse's notes reflect the actions outline in the medication administration record?*
- Obliteration of entries. *Mistakes are common in medical charts. Physicians and nurses are frequently interrupted while writing, and it is not uncommon for them to put in inaccurate information or information meant for another patient's chart. Physicians, nurses, and others are instructed to put a single line through the entry, write "error," and continue with the note. Obliteration of records, such as writing over an entry or using "white out," is never suggested or condoned in a hospital or clinic setting. Such obliterations should be considered suspect.*
- Observations of the nurse conflicting with those of the physician. *Do events occur in one note, but not in the other? Are timed entries in one note completely ignored or omitted in another's note?*
- Changes in the style of note writing. *A longer than usual note can be expected at a time when something obvious and untoward occurs, such as a surgical death or misadministration of a blood product. However, an uncharacteristically long note at a time when the effects of a negligent act are not obvious, such as writing a wrong prescription or failing to seek a consultation, may be considered suspicious.*
- Correlations and/or discrepancies between staffing sheets and time cards. *Notes written by staff members who should not have been present at the time of the incident are highly questionable.*
- Entries that are out of chronological order.
- Omitted documentation. *Missing documentation may be detected through interviews with ex-employees.*

The most successful method of determining if a document was actually written on the date declared is to compare the document with other documents known to be written on that date. Handwriting and/or signatures executed on both dates should be utilized.

Q   **When is a missing or destroyed chart not considered spoliation of evidence?**

A   The American Hospital Association recommends that complete patient medical records be retained by health care institutions for 10 years following the latest patient-care usage.[2] After the 10-year period has expired, patient records may be destroyed provided that the institution:

- Is not in violation of any local law
- Retains complete medical records of minors for the period of minority and meets the applicable statute of limitations
- Retains complete records of patients under mental disability in like manner as those of minors
- Abides by the written request for longer preservation by:
  - Any attending or consulting physician;
  - The patient or his lawful agent;
  - Legal counsel for a party having an interest in the patient's record
- Permanently retains basic information, such as admission and discharge dates, names of responsible physicians, records of diagnosis and operations, surgical reports, pathology reports, and discharge resumes, for all other records that are destroyed.

Q   **What should be done when you find evidence of chart tampering?**

A   When a reviewer of a medical chart is suspicious of chart tampering, the following actions should be taken:

- All suspected entries should be marked as such in a copy of the file
- The original chart should be reviewed for consistency of copy and contents

---

[2]*See* "Preservation of Medical Records in Health Care Institutions," *Technical Advisory Bulletin,* American Hospital Association, 1975.

- An analysis of the suspect entry should be written by the reviewer describing why the entry appears to be tampered with
- The attorney should be notified of the suspicions immediately, and, if indicated, the original chart should be analyzed by a forensic document expert

CHAPTER 28

Malpractice Basics

It is beyond the scope of this book to explain all the nuances of malpractice litigation. Instead, this chapter will give the reader an overview of the basics of malpractice litigation that will help when reviewing a medical record.

Q

A *Medical malpractice* is a professional misconduct or an unreasonable lack of skill. Negligence is the predominant theory of liability in a medical malpractice case.

Q **What is medical malpractice?**

   Medical malpractice comes in many forms, and, even though it would be instructive, a complete list of these forms would be too long. A brief list of the types of medical malpractice would include misdiagnosis, improper treatment, failure to treat, delay in treatment, failure to perform appropriate follow-up, failure to call an appropriate consultant, failure to get informed consent, prescription errors, and treatment inconsistent with the norms of a represented specialty.

Q **What are necessary conditions for a malpractice suit?**

A Our constitution guarantees that anyone can sue to settle a perceived wrong. The courts require that a malpractice claim meet specific criteria to be successful. Specifically, there are four elements that must be proven:

- The physician had a duty to treat the patient.
- A standard of care for treatment of the patient's condition existed, and the physician failed to meet the standard of care.
- The patient suffered damage or injury.
- The physician's failure to meet the standard of care caused the injury to the patient.

Q   **What is meant by a "duty to treat?"**

A   The physician-patient relationship is a contractual relationship that creates a legal duty on the part of the physician to care for the patient. Ordinarily, this relationship is established when the patient seeks medical care and the physician voluntarily agrees to provide that care. In most nonemergent instances, the physician has a choice of whether he wants to treat a patient or not. However, once a physician agrees to treat a patient, the physician has assumed a duty to treat the patient with that degree of skill, care, and diligence possessed or exercised by competent and careful physicians in a similar situation.

Entering a physician's office is a traditional way to seek medical care. Generally, this will invoke the physician-patient relationship and the physician's duty of reasonable care. Less traditional ways of seeking medical care are becoming the norm of late.

A physician has a duty to treat a patient if one of the following conditions exists:

- A physician has established physician-patient relationship based on prior office or hospital visits.
- A patient presents himself to an emergency department where the physician, as a condition of medical staff membership, must take call for an emergency department.
- The physician or his group has a contract with an insurance company or other entity accepting responsibility to care for a group that includes the patient.
- The physician is contacted by phone or arrives at the scene of an accident where the patient has need of immediate medical assistance.
- The patient has made an appointment and come to the physician's office.

Q   **What is a "breach of the standard of care?"**

A   In a malpractice case, the plaintiff must prove that the treating
physician made a mistake. If the physician were to successfully
demonstrate that he had met the acceptable standard of care,
then there would be *no malpractice*. The mistake that the physician makes must be one that a reasonable and prudent physician
would not have made under the same or similar circumstances.
Each practitioner must provide a quality of care sufficient to meet
the criterion known as the "standard of care." The standard dictates that the care provided be, at minimum, equivalent to that
of an average practitioner in the physician's specialty.

The standard of care, unfortunately, can be a "moving target."
In fact, the standard of care for a specific treatment or procedure
may vary from case to case according to the testimony of the
medical experts. Unfortunately, the courts recognize no over-
arching governing body that defines what the standard of care is
for any particular case.

The complex and rapidly changing nature of medical care does
not allow the legislature to create a standard of care, as they have
done in other areas such as operating a small business, a motor
vehicle, or paying income taxes. While medical practice standards exist in texts and in consensus statements from various
specialty societies, those texts and statements are not always
unanimous in their recommendations. Therefore, the courts have
delegated the establishment of medical standards to members of
the medical profession. An *expert witness* establishes a standard
for medical care in the instant case and offers an opinion on
whether the defendant's conduct met this standard.

Q   **What is the importance of "foreseeability" in the
determination of the standard of care?**

A   An important part of demonstrating a breach of the standard of
care is to prove that the bad outcome was foreseeable. Logically,
if a reasonable and prudent person cannot predict that his
actions will result in harm, he cannot be held liable for that harm.
The concept of foreseeability is the basis of every negligence
claim. *Foreseeability,* as it applies to medical malpractice, implies
that any reasonable and prudent health care professional in the

same situation would have been able to predict the poor outcomes of his actions or omissions, and avoided them. The medical experts in a malpractice case must demonstrate to the jury how the poor outcome was foreseeable, and what the physician or nurse could have done differently that would have avoided the poor outcome.

Q   What are the "schools of practice" and "locality" rules?

A   Obtaining expert testimony can be the most difficult part of medical malpractice litigation. This difficulty arises from reluctance by members of a professional group to testify against their colleagues. However, non-colleague health practitioners (i.e., competitors) are fair game. Historically, allopathic physicians (MDs) have been happy to label osteopaths (DOs), homeopaths, or chiropractors as incompetent or dangerous practitioners. The osteopaths, homeopaths, and chiropractors were happy to reciprocate. These rivalries did not create an environment of objective evaluation that was necessary for a fair trial. This led the courts to use the legal doctrines of the "school of practice" and the "locality rule" as the basis for qualifying a person as an expert witness.

Schools of Practice

The school of practice distinctions predate modern medical training and certification. At one time medical practitioners were divided into chiropractors, homeopaths, allopaths, osteopaths, and several other schools based on different philosophical and psychological beliefs. State legislatures did not discriminate among these different schools of healing; that is, all schools of healing were considered equally effective under the law. Therefore, judges were reluctant to allow litigation to be used to attack an "approved" school. Except for chiropractors, allopathic practices (and osteopaths using primarily allopathic methods) have driven out the other schools of medical practice. The courts retain the traditional school of practice rule when they refuse to allow physician experts to question chiropractic care or chiropractors to testify in cases with physician defendants.

The school of practice rule is now applied to the differentiation of physicians into self-designated specialties (self-designated because few state licensing boards recognize specialties or limit physicians' right to practice the specialties in which they have been trained). The relevance of the specialty qualifications of an expert witness depends on whether the case concerns procedures and expertise that are intrinsic to the specialty or general medical knowledge and techniques that are common to all physicians. This dichotomy is reflected in strategies for expert testimony. Whether the parties to the lawsuit will stress the specialty or general knowledge depends on the qualifications of the expert that each has retained. For example, a cardiologist could testify against an emergency department physician if the testimony was limited to the knowledge or a procedure that was common to both, such as performing cardiopulmonary resuscitation. However, a pathologist could not testify against a gastroenterologist on the appropriate diagnosis and treatment of a patient with cirrhosis of the liver.

The Locality Rule

In many parts of the country, the scarcity of specialty physicians and lack of access to tertiary-care centers, especially outside of urban centers, created a gulf between the typical medical care rendered to patients in urban and rural areas. Physicians (and others) in the rural areas feared that they would be unfairly judged by expert witnesses only familiar with the practice of medicine in large university medical centers. For example, when a physician who practiced in a university hospital in a large metropolitan area would testify against a practitioner in a small rural town that lacked access to even the most basic of tertiary-treatment facilities, the university physician might find that the rural physician's diagnosis and treatment had deviated from the medical standards practiced in the university medical center, even though the rural physician had practiced the best medicine allowable in those circumstances. Therefore, a rule was created that assured that a physician's competence would be determined by comparison with the other physicians in the same community or, at least, in similar neighboring communities.

A strict interpretation of this rule, in addition to the natural reluctance of physicians to testify against their colleagues, tends to prevent expert testimony in most malpractice cases. As a result, this rule is not enforced in most courts. In some states, the locality rule has been reintroduced in an attempt to decrease the amount of malpractice litigation, especially in rural areas that are medically underserved.

What is causation?

Causation is also referred to as the proximate cause, the causal connection, or the "but for" principle. If the patient has suffered an injury for which he claims compensation, proximate cause must be demonstrated. Proximate cause consists of finding the "causation in fact." The determination of proximate cause depends upon whether the evidence shows that the results of misconduct are reasonably foreseeable. Therefore, in addition to showing the jury where the defendant physician made a error, the plaintiff's counsel has to show how the physician's actions or omissions, which deviated from the standard of care, directly caused an injury to the patient or that those actions deprived the plaintiff of a significant chance of avoiding or minimizing the harm.

What are damages in a malpractice case?

In order to succeed in a malpractice case, the plaintiff has to show what "damages" resulted from the physician's mistakes. If the plaintiff is unable to demonstrate damages, there is no proof of medical negligence.

The things that normally constitute *damages* in a medical malpractice claim are substantial physical or psychological injuries and/or substantial financial losses. The following are examples of physical injuries:

- Death
- Disability
- Deformity
- Severe and prolonged pain

The following will rarely (if ever) be the kind of damages that will support a medical malpractice claim:

- Mental distress
- Outrage for indifferent care
- Minor pain
- Fear of disease

The commission of an act that could have caused the patient harm, but did not, is insufficient to prove negligence.

Claims for special damages are usually divided, by the "trier of fact," into economic losses and noneconomic losses.

Past and Future Economic Loss

Examples of economic losses include loss of ability to work, loss of future earnings, and loss of money due to medical expenses. Often, economists or other financial experts are necessary to calculate and present these damages.

Past and Future Noneconomic Loss

Some examples of noneconomic losses include loss of sexual function, loss of consortium, physical pain, disfigurement, and emotional suffering.

Q   **Do all instances of medical malpractice result in a malpractice suit?**

A   In 1991, a now famous study was published by Harvard University Researchers.[1] In this study the medical records of 31,424 patients admitted to New York State hospitals were screened for episodes of negligence and injuries that were caused by medical care. Brennan et al. later extrapolated these findings to all admissions to hospitals in the state of New York.[2] A total of 98,607 adverse events were projected (3.5% of hospitalizations), 27,179 negligent adverse events (1% of hospitalizations), and 3,570 malpractice claims (0.1%).

   This study and others[3] revealed the following surprising facts:

- During the course of standard medical management, there is a substantial amount of avoidable injury to patients.
- Many of these avoidable injuries are the result of substandard care.
- Malpractice litigation infrequently compensates patients injured by medical negligence
- Malpractice litigation rarely identifies or holds providers accountable for their substandard care
- The researchers admit they could *not* find negligence in most cases where legal claims were actually filed.

   It can be concluded from these data that most cases of negligence are not pursued by patients or their surviving family members.

---

[1]T. A. Brennan et al., "Incidence of Adverse Events and Negligence in Hospitalized Patients. Results of the Harvard Medical Practice Study I," *N Engl J Med,* 324, 1991, pp. 370–376.

[2]T. A. Brennan et al., "Relation Between Negligent Adverse Events and the Outcomes of Medical-Malpractice Litigation," *N Engl J Med,* 335, 1996, pp. 1963–1967.

[3]A. R. Localio et al., "Relation Between Malpractice Claims and Adverse Events Due to Negligence. Results of the Harvard Medical Practice Study III," *N Engl J Med,* 325, 1991, pp. 245–251.

Q   **If it's not for negligence, why do people sue their physicians?**

A   Malpractice suits don't necessarily occur because of negligence or even a bad outcome, but because of bad relationships between providers and patients. One study[4] documented that "poor relationships with providers before the injury" were responsible for 53% of calls to a plaintiff attorney's offices. Other important causes for calling an attorney mentioned in this study were explicit recommendations by health care providers to seek legal counsel and the impression, held by the patient, of not being kept informed by the providers.[5,6,7]

Q   **What is the natural history of a malpractice suit?**

A   According to a National Academy of Sciences study, only 1 in 8 cases presented to medical malpractice attorneys are pursued.[8] The following is a list of the most common reasons for dropping cases:

- Medical negligence could not be demonstrated.
- Financial recovery is expected to be too small.
- The statute of limitations has lapsed.

This study demonstrates that most potential medical malpractice claims lack the merits of a successful case. Attorneys are unlikely to be willing to pursue such cases. Most of the medical malpractice cases that are pursued are settled before trial. In a study[9] completed by the General Accounting Office of the U.S.

---

[4]L. I. Huycke and M. M. Huycke. "Characteristics of Potential Plaintiffs in Malpractice Litigation. *Ann Intern Med,* 120(9), 1994, pp. 792–798.

[5]W. Levinson et al., "Physician-Patient Communication: The Relationship with Malpractice Claims Among Primary Care Physicians and Surgeons," *JAMA,* 277, 1997, pp. 553–559.

[6]G. B. Hickson et al., "Factors That Prompted Families to File Medical Malpractice Claims Following Perinatal Injuries," *JAMA,* 268, 1992, pp. 1413–1414.

[7]H. B. Beckman et al., "The Doctor-Patient Relationship and Malpractice Lessons from Plaintiff Depositions," *Arch Intern Med,* 155, 1994, p. 543.

[8]*Beyond Malpractice: Compensation for Medical Injuries,* National Academy of Sciences, Institute of Medicine, Washington, DC, March 1978.

[9]U.S Congress, General Accounting Office, *Medical Malpractice: A Framework for Action,* U.S. Government Printing Office, Washington, DC, GAO/HRD-87-73, May 1987.

Congress, the following reasons for the pre-trial settlements were found:

- The case lacked legal merit.
- The plaintiffs dropped the case.
- The defense attorney felt the case was indefensible.
- The defense attorney feared that an emotionally compelling plaintiff might sway the sympathies of a jury, despite the lack of evidence for negligence.
- The defense attorney feared that the defendant would make a poor witness. *He or she believed that the jury might be swayed by their anger at the defendant or their impression that the defendant is incompetent based on his looks and speech.*
- The attorney for the defense decided to settle when he or she felt that the potential for financial loss was greater at a trial than with a negotiated settlement.

Q   **Do other legal duties arise from the physician-patient relationship?**

A   A suit for negligence, based on the precept of foreseeability, can extend to injuries that the patient causes to a third party if the treating physician could anticipate that harm. The courts have held that foreseeable injuries that a patient may cause to others obligate the physician to warn those that may be harmed; that is, it engenders in the physician a "duty to warn." This duty can arise from both physical and psychiatric diseases.

Some examples of physical diseases that invoke a duty to warn include:

Communicable Diseases

Patients with serious communicable diseases, such as tuberculosis, syphilis, HIV, etc., have a foreseeable chance to infect sexual partners or those they live with.

Accidents

Medical conditions such as dementias and epilepsy and medications that can cause drowsiness, loss of coordination, or loss of consciousness all have a foreseeable danger to the patient when driving or at work. These medical conditions also pose a preventable hazard to other drivers, pedestrians, or coworkers. The physician has a duty in these cases to warn the patient, the family, employers, or appropriate licensing agencies.

Psychiatric Diseases

In the case of psychiatric diseases, the physician has a duty to warn others if the patient expresses a desire or intention to harm others or himself. The courts have held that, in the situation that the patient poses a threat to a third party, the physician's duty to the third party supersedes the physician's obligation to patient confidentiality.[10]

SUMMARY

Malpractice is a tortuous violation of a contract between a patient and a physician. A malpractice suit requires four conditions to exist: a recognized duty to treat, a breach of that duty, a harm caused to the patient by the breach of duty, and a demonstrable causal relationship between the breach of duty and the harm.

Even though medical negligence is frequent, malpractices cases are relatively rare. The motivation for bringing a malpractice case has more to do with the patient's anger toward the physician than it does about a perceived professional negligence. The physician-patient relationship engenders legal duties to the physician. These duties include a duty to treat and a duty to warn. Failure of the physician to meet the standard of care during this treatment can result in negligence. Each malpractice cases require the establishment of the standard of medical care. The standard of care is established during each case by expert witnesses. The "harm" to the patient is determined by reviews of the plaintiff's medical record and by other expert testimony. The majority of complaints brought to plaintiff's attorneys lack the necessary elements of a successful case. Most of the cases that are pursued are settled before trial. The physician also has a duty to warn third parties about the foreseeable danger his or her patient poses to those third parties.

---

[10] *Tarasoff v. the Regents of the University of California et al.,* Calif. Rptr 129, 529 P.2d 553 (Calif. 1974).

CHAPTER 29

Pain and Suffering

Q What is "pain and suffering?"

A "Pain and suffering" is a characterization of the physical or emotional distress resulting from an injury or illness for which a plaintiff can seek monetary compensation. It includes not only physical discomfort, loss of physical abilities (such as the use of a hand or foot), but also any emotional pain a person might suffer (such as worry, anxiety, and fear of future pain or disability), social embarrassment, hopelessness, and anhedonia (i.e., the loss of the pleasures and enjoyment of life).

Q What are the legal implications of pain and suffering?

A When a jury in a malpractice or personal injury case finds for the plaintiff, the judge instructs the jury to award money in the following areas:

- Pecuniary awards (money earmarked for the payment of a plaintiff's medical expenses, lost wages, etc.)
- Nonpecuniary awards such as "punitive damage" and "pain and suffering" awards. *Punitive damages are monetary awards made to the plaintiff as a form of punishment to the defendant. Pain and suffering awards are monetary awards made to the plaintiff. The pain and suffering award is not meant as reim-*

bursement for the medical treatment of illness or injury; rather,
it is a separate part of the settlement. Pain and suffering is
related only to injury or damage claims and represents an
attempt at restitution for distress caused by the illness or
injury.

Though a pain and suffering award is not part of a claim for compensation of medical costs or lost wages, it can constitute a significant portion of jury awards. Even in cases where the medical costs are small, large sums can be awarded to a plaintiff who can persuasively articulate the extent of his pain and suffering.

Several recent decisions by the United States Supreme Court have encouraged judges to carefully review jury awards for punitive damages, while damages for pain and suffering, and other awards that compensate plaintiffs for losses, are treated with deference. In addition, punitive damages have recently become subject to the federal income tax, while pain and suffering awards are not. This can result in juries shifting damage awards to the area of pain and suffering as a way to increase the amount of money the plaintiff gets while still punishing the defendant.

Q

A

What is a pain and suffering report?

It is difficult for one person to appreciate another person's experience of pain for any given injury. However, by presenting the physical manifestations of that pain (e.g., crying, moaning, perspiring, insomnia, agitation, depression, etc.) as well as the limitations that the pain places on the sufferer (e.g., the inability to walk, enjoy sports, or dance at a daughter's wedding), another person begins to understand the extent and complications of the pain.

A common approach to the evaluation of a patient's pain and suffering is to create a "pain and suffering report." The *pain and suffering report* is a structured evaluation of the character, intensity and duration of the pain, as well as the limitations that pain places on the patient.

Who is the author of the pain and suffering report?

While it is ideal for a patient to describe his pain to a jury by himself, it is not always possible. A pain and suffering report is, therefore, helpful when the patient cannot speak for himself, such as when the patient has died or when his injuries have left him physically, emotionally, or cognitively unable to answer questions.

Q   **What is contained in the pain and suffering report?**

A   The following are typical components of a pain and suffering report:

- A summary of the patient's medical history
- A vivid description of the complications and problems experienced by the patient
- A summary of the pertinent parts of the medical record, reporting the plaintiff's pain, its complications, and the medications and therapies used to treat the pain
- A prognosis for pain and physical limitations from expert testimony (if possible)

If the pain and suffering report is developed by an expert witness, then the expert witness may be called later to testify in court as to how the report was created and what data it was based on, and make any explanations that are necessary. The pain and suffering report can help the judge and jury by summarizing lengthy medical records and explaining difficult concepts clearly. In fact, the Federal Rule of Evidence Rule 1006[1] states that contents of voluminous material may be presented by summary. The comments on that rule state that the use of summaries is often the only practical means of presenting the contents of voluminous evidence to the judge and jury.

Q   **What questions should be answered when creating the pain and suffering report?**

A   If it is a "physical type" of pain, the following questions should be asked:

- What type of injury was incurred? *Was the injury physical or emotional? Was the injury a burn, a fracture, laceration, or closed-head trauma?*

---

[1]Rule 1006. Summaries. "The contents of voluminous writings, recordings, or photographs which cannot conveniently be examined in court may be presented in the form of a chart, summary, or calculation. The originals, or duplicates, shall be made available for examination or copying, or both, by other parties at reasonable time and place. The court may order that they be produced in court."

- What was the character of the pain? *Is it pressure-like, burning, lancinating, or throbbing?*
- What brings the pain on? *Is it bending, lifting, walking, or standing for long periods?*
- How severe is the pain?
  - Can it be described using a linear analog scale, where 1 equals almost no pain and 10 is the worst pain you can imagine?
  - Can the severity be characterized using a simile (e.g., "the pain is like having a knife in my back")?
  - Was the intensity of the pain steady, or did it wax and wane?
  - How long was the pain at maximal intensity?
  - How long was the pain at minimal intensity?
- What was the duration of the pain?
  - When did it begin?
  - When did it end?
  - Was it constant or intermittent?
  - How long does an episode of pain last?
- How did the pain affect the patient? *The evaluation of the effect of the pain on the patient's life should examine many areas of his or her life.*
  - How has the pain affected work or employment?
    - Is the patient able to return to work?
    - Can the patient work at the same job?
    - Is the patient able to do all the tasks he or she could before his illness or injury?
    - Is the patient able to work for the same amount of time?
    - Has the pain caused the patient to miss opportunities or promotions?
  - How has the pain affected home or family life?
    - Is the patient able to care for himself or herself?
    - Can the patient cook, clean, bathe himself or herself, shop, or drive a car?
    - Can the patient carry small packages?
    - Is the patient able to enjoy the sports and hobbies he or she enjoyed before the illness or injury?
    - How has the pain limited the patient?
    - Is the patient able to lift his or her children?

- Can the patient play ball with his or her children or take them skating?
  - How has the pain affected relations with spouse or significant other?
    - Is the patient more moody, depressed, or agitated?
    - Can the patient engage in sexual relations?
    - Can the patient relax at home?
    - Has the patient become passive, dependent, or child-like?
    - Does the patient go out with friends, or has he or she become lonely and isolated?
- What treatment does the patient need to deal with the pain?
  - What specialists does the patient see?
    - How many?
    - How often?
    - For how long?
  - What therapies does the patient take?
    - Surgery?
    - Injections?
    - Physical therapy?
    - Medications?
    - Electrical stimulation units?
    - Psychiatric or emotional counseling?
  - What are the effects of the therapy?
    - Improvement or worsening of pain?
    - Time lost and pain from surgeries?
    - Drowsiness or confusion caused by medications?
    - Time, effort, and pain suffered in physical therapy?
    - Time and effort expended in psychotherapy?

If it is an "emotional" type of pain, the following questions should be asked:

- What is the character of the emotional pain?
  - Embarrassment?
  - Humiliation?
  - Paranoia?
  - Fear?
  - Agitation?
  - Confusion?
  - Inability to concentrate?
  - Depression?

- How severe is the emotional pain? *Characterize this by how much it affects the patient.*
- How long does the pain last?
- Did the pain have a discrete duration or is it ongoing?
- Is the pain intermittent or continual?
- Has the pain improved or worsened over time?
- Does the lack of improvement cause the patient anxiety?
- Does the prospect of future pain or disability cause the patient anxiety?
- How has this emotional pain affected the patients life?
- Has the pain affected work or employment? (*See above.*)
- Has the pain affected home or family life? (*See above.*)
- What are the effects of treatment?
  - Improvement or worsening of emotional pain?
  - Time spent in counseling sessions?
  - Adverse medication effects (e.g., sexual side effects, weight gain, or agitation from antidepressants)?

Q **What parts of the medical report are most relevant to the pain and suffering report?**

A The medical record will provide the documentation for the pain and suffering report. The following parts of the medical record provide the most information.

Physician Notes

Any mention of pain in the inpatient or outpatient notes should be copied. Any descriptions of the pain and how it has affected the patient's personal life, family life, or employment should be recorded. Any prescriptions for pain relievers, nonsteroidal anti-inflammatory agents, opiates, anxiolytics, sedatives, sleep aids, anti-depressants, or antipsychotic agents should be recorded; their dose and duration should also be recorded with an indication of how "strong" a medication it is and how high of a dose it is. For example, a prescription for 200 mg of ibuprofen three times a day would indicate a lesser pain than tablets of oxycodone or an injection of morphine sulfate. The reviewer should be on the lookout for statements in the medical record such as the patient *claims* constant pain or the patient *reports* pain in back. These statements could suggest that the physician does not believe the patient is really experiencing pain. They should be recorded and followed up by an attorney in a deposition. Other hints that the physician is unconvinced about the organic nature of the pain are referrals to psychiatrists or counselors, or having the patient undergo a Minnesota Multiphasic Personality Inventory (MMPI). The MMPI is a questionnaire-type psychological test for patients ages 16 and over with 550 true-false statements coded in 4 validity and 10 personality scales that may be administered in both an individual or group format. Among other things, this test helps to detect depression and personality disorders that may make the patient more prone to exaggeration of pain. While depression can be caused by chronic pain and there may be other reasons for a psychiatric or psychological referral, these tests and referrals should be noted and followed up.

Nurse's Notes

Nurse's notes are a rich resource for evidence of pain and suffering. The nurse's notes tend to be more focused on psychosocial issues than the physician's notes. When reviewers examine nurse's notes for evidence to support pain and suffering, they should look for all of the same issues mentioned in the physician's notes above, as well as evaluate the following indicators:

- Sleep quality. *Was the patient awake in the middle of the night writhing in pain, moaning in his or her sleep, or woken up when the pain medication wore off?*
- Interest in food and eating. *Is the patient able to eat, swallow, and hold down food? Can the patient feed him or herself? Can the patient sit up in bed? Has the patient lost his or her appetite? Is the patient nauseated?*
- Ability to perform activities of daily living (ADLs). *The ADLs include dressing, personal hygiene, and grooming and are considered basic functions performed by healthy people. An inability to perform can represent a limitation from pain, a pain medication side effect, or depression. Can the patient complete the ADLs independently? Does the patient have interest in doing them? Does the patient perform the ADLs adequately?*
- Interaction with friends and family. *Is the patient able to interact with visitors? Is he distracted by pain or somnolent from medication? Is the patient depressed and/or uninterested? Is he agitated and combative?*
- Requests for more frequent or higher doses of medication. *How does the patient respond to the medication? Does the patient get complete relief, partial relief, or no relief?*
- Complaints about medication side effects. *Did the patient report side effects from pain medication? Was it somnolence, nausea, vomiting, abdominal pain, or constipation?*

- Vital signs. *Pain can sometimes be inferred from changes in a patient's vital signs such as rapid heart beats, high blood pressure, or rapid respiration.*
- Weight. *Is the patient losing weight due to inability to eat or swallow? Is the patient unable to eat because of nausea from opiates or depression? Is the patient gaining weight because he or she is bed-bound and unable to exercise?*

Pharmacy Record

The *pharmacy record* is the complete list of all the medications that were administered to a patient during a hospitalization or other medical confinement (e.g., in a rehabilitation facility or nursing home). The type of pain medication, the dosage, and frequency can be an indicator of the extent of pain. Therefore, the following information should be abstracted from the plaintiff's pharmacy record:

- What types of analgesics were ordered?
- How high were the doses?
- What frequency were the doses given in?
- For what duration?
- Did the doses of analgesic medication increase, decrease, or remain steady over time?
- Was one type of medication sufficient to manage pain or were multiple medications prescribed?
- Did the types of medication change frequently? *This would indicate difficulties in managing pain or medication side effects.*
- Were medications prescribed for analgesic side effects, such as constipation, nausea, vomiting, or abdominal pain?

If psychological pain is at issue, the pharmacy record should be scrutinized for the following types of medication that may indicate depression, anxiety, insomnia, or delusions:

- Antidepressants
- Antianxiety medications
- Sedatives
- Sleep-inducing agents
- Antipsychotic medications

Specialist or Consultant's Notes

When pain is more severe or lasts longer than the physician expects, the physician may call in a consultant to help evaluate or treat the pain.

Specialists may include orthopedists, neurologists, psychiatrists, cardiologists, plastic surgeons, or the newer pain management specialists. These consultant notes will often explore the issues of pain and limitations more deeply than the average physician's notes. Reviewers should take special note of the following information:

- Orthopedists and rheumatologists will often carefully measure and describe the patient's range of motion, strength, ability to move joints, bend, lift, or flex.
- Cardiologists and pulmonologists describe not only such physiologic measures as cardiac output and forced expiratory volume, but also will record the patient's ability to walk a measured distance, climb stairs, or perform ADLs without chest pain, shortness of breath, or dizziness.
- Plastic surgeons will describe wounds, scars, burns, and other defects. They may also describe needed surgeries to correct the defects or disfigurements. Look for and copy any drawings or photographs of the patient's deformities. While some injuries may be obviously physically painful, such as burns, other injuries may result in psychological pain, such as embarrassment, social phobias, and poor body image, from facial scars, colostomy, mastectomy, or amputation.
- Neurologists may describe pain as either somatic or neuropathic and give some prediction of the prognosis of this pain.
- Pain specialists are often doctors who have trained in either anesthesiology, neurology, or rehabilitation medicine and have gone on to do more training in the specific area of pain management. Their notes should explain most, if not all, of the parameters of pain (as discussed above). Pain specialists' notes often will make a diagnosis, give a prognosis, and offer suggestions for treatment. Proposed treatments may include surgical procedures (such as spinal laminectomy or nerve ablation), pharmalogical treatment (such as opiates or numbing agents such as lidocaine), or psychological counseling (such as behavioral therapy or focused imagery).

The following are other sources of information for a pain and suffering report:

- Interview with patient. An interview with the patient can be an important source of information, when the interviewer is a trained professional who is able to review and record all of the parameters of the pain experience.

- Pain diary. A review of the patient's pain diary can provide important information. A *pain diary* is a document created by the patient that records daily pain experiences, and the limitations on lifestyle that the pain imparts. The diary may report on when the patient's pains occur, what actions bring them on, how long they last, and what are the physical, social, and psychological ramifications of the pain experiences.
- Pain drawing. A *pain drawing* is a personal expression of the patient's pain. The drawing is composed of an outline of a human body (front and back) upon which the patient has drawn areas where he or she feels pain. These pain drawings can be made in multiple colors that represent the various types of pain the patient is feeling (e.g., red is burning pain, blue is lancinating pain, and green is dull achiness). These drawings are made on regular intervals and, thus, represent the changing nature and extent of pain the patient is experiencing.

What is nonorganic pain?

While many patients are truthful in their reports of pain, the following are some of the many issues that can distort the patient's report of pain:

- Concerns about confidentiality
- Problems in communication
- Cognitive disabilities
- Fears of incrimination
- Carelessness
- Secondary gain (e.g., avoiding military service; avoiding work; gaining attention of spouse, family, or friends; and obtaining narcotics or financial compensation).

Is malingering common?

Most physicians assume that all patients' reports of pain are truthful. However, Richard Rogers points out in his book on malingering and deception how naive this assumption can be.[2] He has found that patient malingering is common. To compound this problem, physicians mistakenly believe that their training and experience allow them to objectively evaluate a patient's pain

---

[2]R. Rogers (ed.), *Clinical Assessment of Malingering and Deception*, second edition, Guilford Press, New York, 1997.

and expose malingering. Studies have shown that experienced clinicians can be the poorest judges of patient deception.[3]

With this in mind, the reviewer needs to carefully examine medical charts for clues supporting the assumption that the pain the patient complains of may be a lie. It is the reviewer's job to present all possible motivations for intentional deception, as well as signs of malingering. The following are possible signs of intentional deception:

- A lengthy history of personal injury or workman's compensation claims.
- Incongruence between claimed disability and psychological state. *One would expect that severe disability and/or pain should be accompanied by signs of stress and depression.*
- Unusual or illogical symptoms or complaints (e.g., anesthesia of an entire limb, anesthesia of half of a patient's body, or tooth pain associated with hip flexion, etc.).
- Worsening symptoms upon examination (e.g., the patient only has a limp when being observed by an MD, or only has leg weakness upon examination, but not when climbing stairs into the physician's office).
- Lack of improvement with standard treatment (e.g., when strength training does not improve strength and range of motion exercises result in a decreased range of motion; when pain relievers do not relieve pain).

While these signs are not conclusive of deception, they should be noted by the reviewer. Several of these signs together should prompt further investigation into the suspicion of malingering.

 Q   **What are terms associated with reports of nonorganic pain?**

 A   The following is a list of terms that the pain specialist may use in their discussion if they suspect the patient's level of pain does not fit with observed injuries. These terms may seem repetitive or overlapping. However, they are used frequently in notes of pain specialists and, therefore, should be carefully reviewed.

---

[3]P. Ekman and M. O'Sullivan, "Who Can Catch a Liar?" *American Psychologist*, 46(9), 1991, pp. 913–920.

Somatization

The process by which psychological needs are expressed in physical symptoms; for example, the expression or conversion of anxiety into physical symptoms, a wish for material gain associated with a legal action following an injury, or a related psychological need.

Malingering

Feigning illness or disability to escape work, excite sympathy, or gain compensation. The term is based on DSM IV criteria. In the DSM IV definition of malingering,[4] it stipulates that malingering should be strongly suspected if any combination of the following is noted:

- The presence of an antisocial personality disorder
- Medicolegal context of presentation
- Lack of cooperation during the diagnostic evaluation and in complying with the prescribed treatment regimen
- Marked discrepancy between the plaintiff's claimed stress or disability and the objective findings

MMPI

Abbreviation for Minnesota Multiphasic Personality Inventory test. The MMPI is a questionnaire-type psychological test for patients over the age of 16, with 550 true-false statements coded in 4 validity and 10 personality scales that may be administered in both an individual or group format. This test helps to identify patients with depression or other psychopathologies.

Somatoform Disorder

A group of disorders in which physical symptoms suggesting physical disorders for which there are no demonstrable organic findings or known physiologic mechanisms, and for which there is positive evidence, or a strong presumption that the symptoms are linked to psychological factors; for example, hysteria, conversion disorder, hypochondriasis, pain disorder, somatization disorder, body dysmorphic disorder, or Briquet syndrome.

Somatization Disorder

A mental disorder characterized by presentation of a complicated medical history and of physical symptoms referring to a variety of organ systems, but without a detectable or known organic basis.

---

[4]*Quick Reference to the Diagnostic Criteria from DSM IVTR*, American Psychiatric Association, Washington, DC, 2000, pp. 309–310.

Factitious Disorder

A mental disorder in which the individual intentionally produces symptoms of illness or feigns illness for psychological reasons rather than for environmental goals.

Noogenic Neurosis

A diagnosis in existential psychiatry. It consists of a neurotic symptomatology resulting from existential frustration.

Waddell Sign

Dr. Waddell, an orthopedist, determined that there were five findings on physical examination of the patient that correlated with nonorganic back pain.[5] The following is a list of criteria established by Waddell:

- Cog-wheel release in strength testing
- Pain at the tip of the sacrum
- Whole-leg pain or numbness (nonanatomical distribution)
- Whole-leg giving away (inappropriate weakness)
- Overreaction/exaggeration of symptoms

All of the symptoms listed above can be seen in organic back pain. In fact, most patients with documented organic back pain have at least one of Waddell's criteria. However, patients who have 3 out of 5 of the criteria were much more likely to have nonorganic back pain.

Symptom Magnification Syndrome

A behavioral response to circumstances the sufferer feels he cannot control. The patient seeks to exert control through dramatic reports or displays of symptoms. These behavioral patterns are both self-destructive and tend to be reinforced by social circumstances. That is, the patient accrues a secondary gain through his expressions of pain, such as relief from a job he doesn't enjoy and the receipt of disability payments. The following are some examples of behaviors that are associated with symptom magnification:

- Early widespread complaints with minor trauma
- No indication of any improvement after 1 week
- Progressively worse after 1 or 2 weeks and symptoms spread to new areas

---

[5]G. Waddell and D. C. Turk, "Clinical Assessment of Low Back Pain," in D. C. Turk and R. Melzak (eds.), *Handbook of Pain Assessment*, Guilford Press, New York, 1992, pp. 15–36.

- Extreme tenderness on superficial palpation
- Widespread numbness
- Cog-wheel weakness and strength loss
- General stiffness or rigidity of neck; all ranges limited
- Noncompliance to any suggestion on activation
- Seeks more and more narcotic drugs, or reports that drugs have no effect
- Will not attempt return to work
- Secondary gain apparent (social, vocational, financial)
- Progressively dysfunctional out of proportion to injury
- Personality problems, depression, or hypochondria

CHAPTER 30

Personal Injury Claims

Q
A

What is personal injury?

Personal injury is an area of law that seeks to compensate victims who are harmed by the negligence of others. Personal injury law can also be called tort law. While personal injury suits are usually brought by the injured party, in certain situations, such as in medical negligence or wrongful death cases, a person may bring a personal injury lawsuit on behalf of a loved one.

Q
A

What is a personal injury claim?

Personal injury claims or, more accurately, bodily injury claims are those claims that seek damages for injuries sustained as a consequence of the claimed tort of another. A *tort* is an extra-contractual wrong. Every successful personal injury claim has two principal elements: damages and liability.

- *Damages* are injuries or financial consequences suffered as a result of the defendant's negligence.
- *Liability* is a person or organization's responsibility for a hazard or loss.

To be a successful personal injury claim, the injuries must be caused by the wrongdoing or negligence of another.

Q **What is the theory of liability in personal injury claims?**

A Personal injury claims are based upon the theory that a reasonable and prudent person was harmed by the negligence of another.

Q **What is negligence in personal injury claims?**

A It is generally held, in western law, that individuals have a duty to make reasonable efforts to protect others from harm. For example, property owners cannot allow gross hazards to exist on their property. Situations that present foreseeable accidents and injuries should be corrected in order to make them safe for the public. Open manhole covers, wet and slippery floors, holes in the sidewalk, loose carpeting, unstable railings, and poorly lit stairways are examples of situations that could lead to an injury. The owners of the properties on which these situations exist are liable to the people who may be harmed by these situations. When individuals fail to take reasonable actions to prevent others from foreseeable harm, they are held to be negligent. Negligence of an individual is predicated on the assumption that others would have acted in a prudent and reasonable manner.

Q **What is the reasonable person doctrine?**

A The critical issue in many personal injury cases is how a "reasonable person" was expected to act in the particular situation that caused the injury. A person is negligent when he or she fails to act consistent with the standard of an ordinary reasonable person.

It should be made clear that there is an important distinction between reasonable person and average person. The reasonable person standard is based on how the community judges a reasonable person should behave in the same or similar situation, as opposed to how an average person would behave. The duty is based on the twin elements of rationality and safety. The reasonable person standard does not rely on whether most people actually behave that way. For example, even though it may be common not to report all of one's income to the Internal Revenue Service (IRS), a person who doesn't comply with the tax laws will be subject to penalties if their return is audited. Therefore, even if the average person doesn't report all of his or her income to the IRS, the reasonable person would obey the tax law.

The determination of whether a given person has met the ordinary reasonable person standard is often a matter that is resolved by a jury after presentation of evidence and argument at trial. For example, let's say a person breaks into an electrical utility room that is clearly marked with a sign that states "Caution: High Voltage" and "Danger: Keep Out" and sustains a fatal electrical shock. The property owner may not be liable for this personal injury since the trespasser did not exercise the caution that an ordinary reasonable person would have exercised if put in the same situation.

Liability and damages can be established on several bases.

Negligence

When a case is filed as tort of negligence, the defendant is accused of causing the injury by failing to act as an ordinary and prudent person would have under the same or similar circumstances.

Strict Liability

Under strict liability, a personal injury attorney may also bring charges against a company whose defective product is responsible for an injury. Strict liability only applies to a product when it is being used as intended. Also, persons or companies engaged in using explosives, storing dangerous substances, or keeping dangerous animals can be held strictly liable for harm caused to others as a result of such activities. The theory behind imposing strict liability on those conducting such activities is that these activities pose an undue risk of harm to members of the community. Thus, anyone who conducts such activity does so at his or her own risk and is liable when something goes wrong and/or someone is harmed. Persons or companies may be held strictly liable for certain activities that harm others, even if they have not acted negligently or with wrongful intent.

Intentional Wrong

A tort or wrong perpetrated by one who intends to do that which the law has declared wrong. This is in contrast to negligence where the tortfeasor fails to exercise that degree of care in doing what is otherwise permissible. Intentional wrongs can sometimes be brought as civil claims (i.e., personal injury claims), apart from any criminal charges the defendant may be facing.

Q   **What are the types of personal injury cases?**

A   There are different forums and distinct bodies of law, statutes, and
legal precedents for varying types of personal injury accidents. A
work-related accident is processed by a workers compensation tri-
bunal with its own requirements and prerequisites. Injuries from
car accidents in many states come within the purview of "no-fault
law" and are processed through their own quasi-judicial system of
arbitration determinations. General or public liability accidents
are processed by insurance companies for the entities sued and,
ultimately, by the state and federal courts.

Some types of accidents causing injuries can be processed and
are recoverable in only one forum (to the exclusion of others), while
others afford "two bites of the apple." A carpenter who injures his
hand using a hammer can only recover limited damages from his
employer through the workers compensation forum. However, a
carpenter who is struck on the head by a hammer dropped by the
employee of another contractor can look to both the workers compensation forum and the general liability forum for recovery of
damages. The worker here is not entitled to twice the amount of
damages (i.e., "double dipping"), but rather a sharing or apportion-
ment of recovery from each of the two forums.

A motorist who is injured when his car is struck in the rear and
sustains significant injuries can look to two sources to recover his
damages. He would recover part of his damages from his own car
insurance carrier, under the no-fault law and another part under
the general liability law in making a negligence claim against the
offending motorist who struck him.

The following are the commonest types of personal injury
claims.

Car Accident

Auto accidents, as well as truck and motorcycle accidents, can
result in serious personal injury to those involved in the collision.

Slip and Fall Injury

Also known as premises liability. The owner of the property may
be held liable for injuries that result from foreseeable dangers
that existed on his property.

Medical Malpractice

A suit that arises from personal injuries that occur due to the negligence on the part of a physician or other health care provider whose substandard level of care is the proximate cause of the personal injury.

Job-Related Injury

Injuries that occur to workers and others that are at a jobsite or involved in a job-related activity (e.g., driving a truck between workplaces).

Wrongful Death

When someone is killed as a result of another's negligent actions, the family of the deceased often has grounds for a wrongful death claim.

Nursing Home Abuse

Also known as nursing home neglect. Injuries that occur to nursing home residents as a result of physical abuse, mental abuse, or abandonment.

Defective Product Injury

Also known as products liability case. Injuries that result from defective products, including drug and medical devices.

Injury from Wild or Dangerous Animals

The owners of animals that have a potential to injure others can often be held liable for any personal injury that the animal may cause when their foreknowledge of the animals' vicious propensity is determined by the trier of fact.

Q
A

What is contributory negligence?

Contributory negligence is an element of common law that holds that if a person is injured in part due to his or her own negligence (i.e., his or her negligence contributed to the accident), the injured party would not be entitled to collect any damages (money) from another party who supposedly caused the accident. Under this doctrine, a badly injured person who was only slightly negligent could not win in court against a very negligent defendant. The results of a determination of contributory negligence are often so inequitable that juries tend to ignore them.

What is comparative negligence?

Comparative negligence is a doctrine of comparative fault that is applied in accident cases. The comparative negligence doctrine helps to apportion responsibility for damages based on the negligence of every party directly involved in the accident. In personal injury law, *comparative negligence* refers to the determination of what fault, if any, the complaining party may have in connection with the personal injury that occurred. Comparative negligence laws vary state by state, but, generally, damages recovered may be reduced if the plaintiff is found to be in any way at fault for the accident. In some states, if a jury and judge find that the plaintiff is just as much at fault as the defendant for the injury or accident, no damages will be awarded. The reduction of a plaintiff's award is determined by the percentage of fault that the jury attributes to the plaintiff.

What is an "assumption of risk?"

In most hazardous recreations and sports, individuals voluntarily assume the risk of their actions. The following are common examples of people who voluntarily assume their own risk:

- Skydivers
- Skiers
- Scuba divers
- Player of contact sports
- Car and boat racers
- Passengers on amusement park rides

These activities carry foreseeable risks that the participants are willing to accept. It is common for these individuals to sign a consent form that waives the host's liability in the event that they are injured participating in the activity. Even if no written agreement is signed, implied assumption of risk can sometimes be used as a defense. Choosing to participate, despite the warning, may demonstrate implied assumption of risk.

Can the assertion of diminished mental capacity be a defense for negligence?

A   When an injury occurs due to an accident, the mental capacity of the tort-feasor is usually not taken into account when considering if a defendant is negligent. Juries are directed to consider the actual conduct of the tort-feasor when determining negligence. The following are *not effective* defenses in negligence cases:

- Lack of intelligence
- Poor memory
- Emotional distress
- Drug or alcohol intoxication

Generally, individuals are held to the reasonable person standard despite mental or emotional limitations. Intoxication is not considered an excuse because the individuals chose to drink or use drugs that would foreseeably result in impaired judgment.

Q   **What are "damages" in a personal injury suit?**

A   *Damages* are defined as money awarded in a civil action to a party that has been wrongfully injured by another party. Damages attempt to restore the injured party to the position they were in before the personal injury occurred and are measured by the amount of suffering incurred. Damages can also be recovered for the malicious conduct of the other party.

Q   **Is there a time limit for starting a personal injury suit?**

A   In personal injury law, the *statute of limitations* refers to the period from the time an injury occurs or is discovered to the final date on which a lawsuit can be filed. If the statute of limitations expires before a personal injury lawsuit is filed, the defendant can have the case dismissed for being untimely. It will be up to the defendant to alert the court to a statute of limitations violation. Statutes of limitation can vary from state to state. However, one to three years from the date of harm is a standard limitation. If the harmed individual is not aware of the harm, the statute of limitations may be extended until he or she does become aware or should have become aware. An example of an extension in the statute of limitation is asbestos exposure. Individuals who worked in certain construction industries may have been unwittingly exposed to asbestos during their work lives. The harm this exposure causes was only found out 20–30 years later when the exposed developed malignant mesothelioma. In this case, the statute of limitation would start to run on the date of discovery or manifestation of the patient's diagnosis.

Q   **Does the medical record have a role in personal injury claims?**

A   Medical records have a dimension in personal injury litigation. It is accepted as fact that a patient, when reporting to a physician or hospital (particularly immediately post-incident), will customarily give an accurate history as to the incipient cause of his or her visit and relevant pathologies.

In the course of investigating and evaluating claims for damages, both the attorney representing the injuried party and the attorney representing the person or entity against which the claim is asserted turn to the medical records. Both attorneys hope to either corroborate the basis of the claim or diminish its credibility because of the spontaneity in which the information was recorded.

In the preceding discussion, successful personal injury cases were characterized by the demonstration of both negligence of another person and harm to the plaintiff. Evidence to both substantiate and undermine claims of negligence and harm can be found in the rich vein of the medical record. The following are some examples from the author's experience:

- A child, whose attorney claimed his injury was due to a defective floor, told the triage nurse that he had "tripped over his cat."
- A plaintiff, who alleged injury from a defective stairwell, admitted to a history of frequent cardiac syncope during his admission history.
- A homeowner suing a manufacturer for injuries from using a defective ladder at home admitted in his triage history that he had an "accident at work.".
- A woman, who alleged injury in a retail store, told the emergency medical technician that she fell over a curb in the street.
- A homeowner, who reported severe hand injuries from a "defective" garage door opener, admitted to the emergency

department (ED) physician that he had removed the product's steel safety covering before installation with an acetylene torch.

The above instances are examples of what can be gleaned from a careful reading of the medical record.

Q   **Is determination of the location of an accident an important issue in a negligence case?**

A   A negligence damage claim is predicated, in part, on the *place* the incident (which caused the injury or damage) occurred. The place where the accident occurred often determines who is liable for the injury. Therefore, determining whether the incident occurred on a sidewalk, in the street, or in an automobile will dictate, in part, if the claim has legal merit. Determining the location of the accident or injury is not always easy. The location may not be mentioned at all in the medical record. Sometimes, more than one location is given due to mishearing on the part of the physician or inaccuracies in transcription. Infrequently, less-scrupulous plaintiffs will suffer an injury and later seek a well-insured location, where their chances for monetary recovery are improved. Therefore, the reviewer needs to carefully examine the medical chart for evidence of the location. Reports of the location are more likely to be accurate during the first few hours after the injury, before the patient or family members have had an opportunity to forget, become confused, or consider other less-scrupulous options.

Evidence of location can be found in the medical chart in the following areas:

Ambulance Call Report

Often reports the location of where the patient was found and under what circumstances.

Emergency Department Record

In the first ED interview, the patient will give a lengthy recounting of the accident. This interview will often include information about the exact nature of the accident and its location.

Admission History

As in the ED record, the first interview with the admitting physician tends to be spontaneous and filled with details.

Consulting Physician's Reports

Consultants have the luxury of spending a lot of time interviewing the patient and eliciting a complete history. Their reports tend to be more in-depth and complete.

Q **How does one make a determination of harm or injury from the medical record?**

A The sequence of events following the accident establishes believability to the "trier of fact" (judge or jury), who will ultimately award damages. In the context of the injury sustained or alleged, whether the injured person was conveyed to the hospital by a car, ambulance, or walked in is a significant factor in the investigation of tort claims. These facts should be sought out in the medical chart and entered in the summary report. The extent of harm can usually be determined from the medical record. The following questions should be answered when reading the record:

- How badly was the person injured?
- Did the injuries result from the stated incident or were they preexisting?
- Is the mechanism of injury consistent with the injuries described?
- Is the treatment appropriate for the stated injuries?
- Does the treatment seem excessive or prolonged?
- Did the injuries result in disabilities?
- Is the patient partially or completely disabled?
- Are any resultant disabilities temporary or permanent?
- Are there signs of injury magnification, exaggeration, or fraud?
- Are the appropriate specialists caring for the patient?

Q **How does one determine if the statute of limitations has expired from the medical record?**

A The date of accident can be determined from the medical record. The ED record or admission note will usually state when the accident of injury occurred. In cases of delayed manifestation of harm, such as toxic chemical exposure, asbestosis, medication error, or surgical misadventure, the statute of limitations can be determined from the date of diagnosis of the injury.

Q   **How should comparative negligence be assessed from the medical chart?**

A   As we have seen, *comparative negligence* refers to the determination of what fault, if any, the plaintiff has for his or her own injuries. It is not uncommon in personal injury cases to find that the plaintiff shares some responsibility for his or her injuries. The car accident victim may have been talking on the cell phone while driving, the slip and fall victim may have been intoxicated after leaving a bar on a rainy night, or the victim of a beating may have instigated the fight. Clues to comparative negligence can be found in the medical chart. Like other issues of liability, plaintiffs may want to avoid mentioning this evidence of shared liability when the possibility of financial recovery becomes apparent. Therefore, the medical reviewer should search the earliest recorded interactions between the patient and the health care system. The reviewer should look for the following information.

Ambulance Notes

Look for spontaneous utterances recorded in the ambulance call report (ACR), such as "I was drunk and fell down" or references to alcohol on breath (AOB) or drug use. Does the patient report issues with "too much insulin" or "dizziness" from a new blood pressure medication? Do the EMTs record symptoms that may be associated with intoxication, stroke, or cardiac event? Does the ACR report an assault or suspicions of criminal activity?

Triage Notes

Nurses' triage notes and their other clinical impressions may contain clues that will support further inquiries in one factor of the case or another. For example, the notation "AOB" may underscore the history and even explain causation. Clinical impressions of "lethargy" and "drowsiness" or, conversely, "alert" and "well-oriented" will diminish or underscore the credibility of the patient's recollection of events.

Emergency Department Notes

The ED may be the first interaction of the patient with physicians. The physicians often ask probing questions about the nature and causation of the injuries as a method of determining how severe they are likely to be. Often, the patient will answer truthfully. The ED note should be reviewed for determination of the cause of the injury. Did the patient suffer from weakness or numbness of the legs that led to the slip and fall? Was there evidence of palpitations, chest pain, or shortness of breath before the fall down the stairs? Do the notes reflect a history of seizures in the plaintiff complaining of falling at a work site? A careful review of the ED record may reveal evidence of contributory negligence.

Q

A

What should be asked about physician's office records?

A review of the patient's medical records from his physician's office before and after the accident can reveal important information. The following are some important questions to ask:

- What was the patient's health like before the accident?
- Did he have chronic illnesses?
- Was there any preexisting injuries or disabilities?
- Were there any prior personal injury suits?
- How was the patient employed prior to the accident?
  - Was he in a job where he was exposed to respiratory irritants or toxic chemicals?
  - Was he exposed to repetitive trauma of the hands, legs, or back?
  - Did he handle vibrating tools or equipment (e.g., drills, jackhammers, or sanders)?
  - Was he employed in hard physical labor?
- Were there prior worker's compensation claims?
- Were there any prior neurologic or psychiatric illnesses?
- Did the patient have prior testing, such as a CT or MRI scan, that may have documented preexisting injuries?
  - What were the complaints that prompted these exams?
  - Are the previous complaints similar or identical to the current complaints?
- Did the patient participate in contact sports?

- Did the patient have physically dangerous hobbies or interests (e.g., skydiving or motorcycle racing)?
- Was there prior military service?
  - What did the patient do while in the military?
  - Were there any accidents claimed while in training or during combat service?
  - Was there any exposure to toxic chemicals or biologicals?
  - Were there any disabilities claimed from military service?
- Was there any medical therapy?
  - Do the physician's notes reflect goals for the therapy?
  - Do the physician's notes reflect steady improvement in pain, mobility, or ability to work?
  - Do the physician's notes reflect lack of improvement with therapy?
  - Is the therapy changed or is it continued despite lack of improvement?
  - How long does the therapy last?
  - Is the patient compliant with the therapy?
  - Does the patient attend all therapy sessions?
  - Does the patient fill prescriptions?
  - Does the physician document disabilities?
  - Are any disabilities characterized as temporary or permanent?

Q **What should be asked about physical therapy records?**

- Were goals stated for physical therapy?
  - Who set the goals (therapist or physician)?
  - Was treatment progress measured against goals?
- Do the patient's complaints at the therapist's office match the complaints at the physician's office?
- Did the therapist document the patient's behavior, attitude, or physical condition during the visits?
- Is there a consistent application of treatment modalities during therapy? Or does it change frequently and illogically?
- How frequently was the therapy recommended?
- How frequently did the patient participate in his therapy?
- How long was therapy given?
- Are there changes in the frequency of therapy visits over time?

- Were attempts made at teaching the patient to do the therapy at home?
- Did the therapist document any improvement in the patient's condition over time (e.g., mobility, range of motion, exercise tolerance, or pain level)?
- Did the therapist document any injuries that occurred after the accident, but during the therapeutic period?

Glossary of Malpractice Terms

Abandonment.   Desertion or willful forsaking of a patient. Forgoing medical duties.

Action.   A lawsuit brought in court. A formal complaint within the jurisdiction of a court of law.

***Ad Damnum* Clause (Latin).**   *Ad Damnum* refers to the parts or sections of a petition that speak to the damages that were suffered and claimed by the plaintiff. The *Ad Damnum* part of a petition will usually suggest an amount in dollars that the plaintiff asks the court to award. An *Ad Damnum* clause prevents the plaintiff from stating how much money he is suing for. This eliminates some of the sensationalism in a trial.

Advanced directive.   A document that expresses the wishes of a person, should they become terminally ill or have a serious accident. (See also living will and health care proxy.)

Affirmative defense.   In a defendant's case, it is the raising of facts and allegations to defeat the prosecution's case.

Age of majority.   The age one becomes a legal adult and gains full legal rights, such as the right to vote.

Agent.   One who is permitted to act for or in place of someone else. A person who has received the power to act on behalf of another. The acts performed by the agent have the power of attorney that binds the other person, as if he himself were making the decisions. The person who is being represented by the agent is referred to as the "principal."

Aggravated damages.   Special and highly exceptional damages awarded by a court where the circumstances of the tortuous conduct have been particularly humiliating or malicious toward the plaintiff or victim.

Answer.   The response to a pleading, addressing the merits of a legal case.

Assault.   A threat or use of force on another that reasonably makes that person fear bodily harm. Also, the touching of another person with intent to harm, without that person's consent.

Assumption of risk.   A plaintiff who voluntarily enters into a risky situation, knowing the risk, cannot recover damages. This does not include a risk different from or greater than the risk normally involved in the situation.

Acquittal.   Where a jury finds a defendant not guilty.

Battery.   The use of force on another resulting in harmful contact; a criminal act.

Best evidence rule.   Requires that for a document to be entered into evidence, it must be the original document, unless the original document is unavailable. If the unavailability of the original is adequately explained, copies or secondary evidence of what was in the original are sometimes allowed.

Bench.   In a courtroom, it is the seat occupied by a judge. Also, a judge in court session.

Breach.   An infraction or violation of the law.

Breach of duty.   Any violation or omission of a legal or moral duty. The neglect or failure to fulfill, in a just and proper manner, the duties of an office or fiduciary employment.

Breach of contract.   The failure to do what one promised to do under a contract. Proving a breach of contract is a prerequisite of any suit for damages based on a contract.

Breach of trust.   Any act or omission, on the part of the trustee, that is inconsistent with the terms of the trust agreement or the law of trusts. A prime example is the redirecting of trust property from the trust to the trustee.

Burden of proof.   In litigation, a party's duty to prove a disputed assertion to succeed or move on in a legal proceeding.

Captain of the ship doctrine.   Imposes liability on a principal for the acts of his agents. For example, a surgeon in charge of an operation may be successfully sued for negligence of his assistants during the period when those assistants are under his control, even though those assistants are also employees of the hospital.

Causation.   The act by which an effect is produced. The act that was the proximate cause of the harm in a case.

Cause in fact.   The particular cause that produces an event and, without which, the event would not have occurred. The courts commonly referred to this as the "but for" rule: "The injury to an individual would not have happened but for the conduct of the wrongdoer."

Cause of action.   The reason a lawsuit may be brought to court. The specific grievance or violation of rights that gives grounds for a legal action. A group of facts that give rise to the rights of action; a lawsuit.

Capacity.   Individual's ability or competence, especially in terms of responsibility for committing a crime or ability to execute a legal document (e.g., give consent).

Claim.   The assertion of a right to money or property.

Comparative negligence.   A rule of law applied in accident cases to determine responsibility and damages based on the negligence of every party directly involved in the accident.

Competency.   In the law of evidence, the presence of those characteristics or the absence of those disabilities that render a witness legally fit and qualified to enter into contracts, sign documents, or create other written evidence.

Compos mentis [Latin].   Sound of mind. Having use and control of one's mental faculties.

Consent.   A voluntary agreement by a person in the possession of sufficient mental capacity to make an intelligent choice to do something proposed by another.

Continuous treatment doctrine.   Under this doctrine, the time in which to bring a medical malpractice action is stayed when the course of treatment, which includes wrongful acts or omissions, has run continuously and is related to the same original condition or complaint.

Contributory negligence.   A doctrine of common law that states if a person was injured in part due to his/her own negligence (i.e., his or her negligence "contributed" to the accident), the injured party would not be entitled to collect any damages (money) from another party who supposedly caused the accident. Under this rule, a badly injured person who was only slightly negligent could not win in court against a very negligent defendant. The results of a determination of contributory negligence are often so unfair that juries tend to ignore them. Many states do not follow this system.

Culpa lata [Latin for "gross negligence"].   More than just simple negligence. It includes any action or an omission in reckless disregard of the consequences to the safety or property of another.

Damages.   The money that is sought from a defendant by a plaintiff in a lawsuit, and is awarded to the plaintiff as a remedy for some injury or wrongdoing.

Decedent.   A dead person; in particular, one who has died recently.

Decision.   A determination made after considering the facts and law, in a legal context; a determination of a judicial nature.

Deep pocket.   A person or corporation of substantial wealth and resources from which a claim can be made.

Defendant.   A person who is charged with a crime in a criminal case or has a claim against them in a civil case.

Deponent.   A person who testifies at a deposition.

Deposition.   A pretrial statement given under oath in front of a court reporter, but without a judge present. A deposition can be used as evidence in a trial.

Detrimental reliance.   A party may be obligated by a promise when he or she knew or should have known that the promise would induce the other party to rely on it to his detriment, and the other party was reasonable in so relying. Recovery may be limited to the expenses incurred or the damages suffered as a result of the promisee's reliance on the promise. Reliance on a gratuitous promise made without required formalities is not reasonable.

Discovery.   A pretrial process in which each side requests relevant information and documents from the other. Parties must provide the requested information or documents or show good cause to the court why they should not have to do so.

Due process of law.   Procedural due process: A course of official actions or a proceeding that follows established rules and principles.

Duty.   A legal or moral obligation. An obligation that one has by law or contract. An obligation that the law recognizes to comport to a particular standard of conduct toward another.

Durable power of attorney.   A document in which one person (the principal) gives authority to another to act on his or her behalf should the principal become unable to do so. The designated individual is known as an attorney-in-fact, although the person need not be a lawyer.

Durable power of attorney (for health care).   A document in which the principal appoints an agent to make health care decisions. It contains the wishes of the principal regarding the medical treatment he wishes or does not wish to receive.

Emergency doctrine.   The rule that exempts people from the ordinary standard of reasonable care if that person acted instinctively to help out someone who needed emergency assistance.

Emergency Medical Treatment and Active Labor Act.   Once it is established that a patient appeared at a hospital's emergency department with an emergency medical condition, or when an individual has been diagnosed as presenting an emergency medical condition, the hospital must provide that treatment necessary to prevent the material deterioration of the individual's condition or provide for an appropriate transfer to another facility. The hospital will be liable under the Emergency Medical Treatment and Active Labor Act either if it fails to detect the nature of the emergency condition as a result of a disparate screening or, if the hospital detects the emergency condition, by failing to stabilize the condition prior to releasing the patient.

Emotional distress.   The legal claim of pain and suffering that affect the mind as the result of a physical injury; the injury can be recoverable in monetary compensation.

Evidence.   The means by which an alleged matter of fact is established or disproved.

Exonerate.   To free one from responsibility.

Expert.   Someone who, through education or experience, has gained enough knowledge of a particular subject so that he or she could form an opinion that one without that knowledge could not.

Expert witness.   One who, by reason of education or specialized experience, possesses superior knowledge of a subject about which persons having no particular training are incapable of forming an accurate opinion or deducing a correct conclusion.

Express warranty.   A warranty created by the express or overt words of the seller.

Federal Tort Claims Act.   An important issue in medical malpractice cases. It authorizes civil actions for damages against the United States for personal injury or the termination of life caused by the negligence of a government employee under circumstances in which a private person would be liable under the law of the state in which the negligent act or omission occurred.

Finding of fact.   What the court (judge or jury) determines the actual facts are in the case after listening to the evidence.

Foreseeability.   Being such as may be reasonably anticipated, as in "a foreseeable problem." In a negligence suit, foreseeability may imply a duty to act.

Guardian.   One who has been entrusted by the law for the care of another person or for his estate or for both.

Health care directive.   Any statement made by a competent individual about preferences for future medical treatment in the event that he is unable to make decisions at the time of treatment.

Health care proxy.   The person that someone appoints to make health care decisions in the event that the person is unable to express his or her wishes due to illness or incapacitation.

Hearsay rule.   A rule of evidence that generally prohibits a person from providing testimony based upon what that person has been told or learned secondhand. Instead, the rules of evidence favor testimony based upon a person's own observations.

Implied consent.   Consent indicated by signs and actions or lack of objection.

Incapacity.   To lack the legal, physical, or intellectual ability to stand trial, give consent, make a valid will.

Incompetency.   Lacking legal qualifications or physical, intellectual, or fitness to perform required duty.

Indemnification.   The act of compensating for loss or a damage.

Indemnify.   To reimburse a loss that someone has suffered because of another's act or default.

Independent contractor.   One who is hired to complete a specific project but is free to do that work as he or she wishes;

an independent contractor is not an employee, thus cannot sue an employer for a wrongful act or injury suffered on the job.

Indicia.   Distinctive signs or indications that support a belief; similar to circumstantial evidence.

Informed consent.   A person's agreement to allow something to happen (such as surgery) that is based on a full disclosure of risks and benefits needed to make an intelligent decision.

In loco parentis **[Latin for "in place of a parent"].**   A person or institution that assumes parental rights and duties for a minor.

Intentional tort (willful tort or intentional wrong).   A tort or wrong perpetrated by one who intends to do that which the law has declared wrong as contrasted with negligence in which the tort-feasor fails to exercise that degree of care in doing what is otherwise permissible.

Interrogatories.   Written questions developed by one party's attorney for the opposing party. Interrogatories must be answered in writing, under oath, and within a specific period of time.

Insurance.   A system of protection in which one party agrees to guarantee another against specific damages or losses.

Joint and several liability.   The sharing of liability both individually and collectively, as in a negligence suit.

Judgment.   The final decision of the court resolving the dispute and determining the rights and obligations of the parties.

Jurisdiction.   The sphere of authority to rule on questions of law; authority to govern or legislate.

Jury trial.   A judicial examination of fact or law whose outcome is decided by a jury.

Learned intermediary doctrine.   Provides that a pharmaceutical manufacturer's duty to provide an adequate warning for prescription drugs runs *to the physician*, not the patient. Generally, a prescription drug manufacturer may satisfy its duty to the user of the drug by giving an adequate warning to the user's physician, and not to the user himself or herself.

Although a manufacturer's duty to warn runs to all foreseeable users of the product, in some cases a manufacturer "may be absolved from blame because of justified reliance upon a middleman." *MacDonald v. Ortho Pharmaceutical Corp.*, 394 Mass. 131, 135 (1985) (quotation omitted).

Legal duty.   An obligation resulting from a law or legal contract.

Liability.   A person or organization's extent of responsibility for a hazard or loss.

Litigants.   Participants in a lawsuit, either as plaintiffs or defendants.

Litigation.   A lawsuit. The process of using a court to resolve a problem or seek remedy for a harm.

Living will.   A document wherein a person states his or her intention to refuse medical treatment and release health care providers from liability if the person becomes terminally ill and is unable to state his or her refusal.

Locality rule.   A rule that states that a physician is only required to possess and apply the knowledge and use the skill and care that is ordinarily used by reasonably well-qualified physicians in the locality, or similar localities, in which he or she practices.

Lost chance doctrine (or loss of chance).   In medical malpractice actions, refers to the injury sustained by a patient whose medical providers negligently deprived the patient of a chance to survive or recover from a health problem, or where the malpractice lessened the effectiveness of treatment or increased the risk of an unfavorable outcome to the patient.

Malfeasance.   A wrongful act of some sort.

Malice.   The intent to commit a wrongful act without justification for doing so.

Malpractice.   A misconduct, lack of skill, or unreasonable mistake in a professional capacity, usually applied to physicians, lawyers, or accountants. Stated alternatively, malpractice is a violated duty that causes harm.

Mitigate.   To make less severe.

Motion.   A request to a court for an action.

Neglect.   The failure to act, provide care, or perform a duty that should be performed, due to either law or legal contract.

Negligence.   The failure to act in a manner that could be considered reasonable and/or prudent under the circumstances. Negligence is committing an act that a person exercising ordinary care would not do under similar circumstances definition or the failing to do what a person exercising ordinary care would do under similar circumstances.

***Non compos mentis* [Latin for "not of sound mind"].** Idiocy, insanity, and incompetence.

Notice.   Formal notification of a legal proceeding.

Ostensible agency.   A form of the implied agency relationship created by the actions of the parties involved, rather than by written agreement or document.

Out-of-court settlement.   An agreement between two litigants to settle a matter privately before the court has rendered its decision.

Pain and suffering.   The emotional and physical injuries for which a person may seek recovery in a tort action.

Party.   A person or entity that is the plaintiff or defendant in a lawsuit.

Personal injury.   The area of law that seeks to protect victims who are harmed by the action or inaction of another person or entity.

Plaintiff.   The complaining party in a civil lawsuit.

Pleadings.   The allegations of facts supporting the claims and defenses asserted in a lawsuit.

Power of attorney.   A document that gives one person the right to act for another. The power of attorney may be general or specific, such as a "medical power of attorney."

Preponderance of the evidence.   The level of proof required in a civil case; one side's case must simply be considered more provable than the other's. It is the lowest level of proof.

Prima facie **[Latin for "on its face" or "at first view"].**   At first glance; as things appear on the first impression.

Privileged communication.   A communication that is protected from forced disclosure by legal privilege.

Proximate cause.   A cause that immediately precedes and produces the effect and is distinguished from the remote, mediate, or predisposing cause. That which in ordinary natural sequence produces a specific result with no independent disturbing agencies intervening.

Proxy.   A person or organization with the power to represent or serve in the place of another. Proxy can also refer to the document that gives such authorization.

Prudent patient standard.   A standard that states that a reasonably prudent patient under similar circumstances would not have consented to the treatment if informed of such material fact or facts.

Punitive damages.   Special and highly exceptional damages ordered by a court against a defendant where the act or omission that caused the suit, was of a particularly heinous, malicious, or high-handed nature. Where awarded, they are an exception to the rule that damages are to compensate, not to punish. The exact threshold of punitive damages varies from jurisdiction to jurisdiction. In some countries and in certain circumstances, punitive damages might even be available for breach of contract cases but, again, only for the exceptional cases where the court wants to give a strong message to the community that similar conduct will be severely punished. Punitive damages are most common in intentional torts such as rape, battery, or defamation. Some jurisdictions prefer using the term "exemplary damages," and there is an ongoing legal debate whether there is a distinction to be made between the two and even with the concept of aggravated damages.

Question of fact.   An issue involving the resolution of a factual dispute and, hence, within the province of the jury, in contrast to a question of law.

Question of law.   A question concerning the legal effect to be given an undisputed set of facts. An issue that involves the application or interpretation of a law and, hence, within the province of the judge and not the jury.

Reasonable care.   The care that most reasonable people would be expected to take under a certain set of circumstances.

Reasonable person test.   A test applied to the facts and particular circumstances in which the mind of the defendant should be exercised.   This test assumes normal circumstances. "Negligence is the omission to do something which a reasonable [person], guided upon considerations which ordinarily regulate the conduct of human affairs, would do or doing something which a prudent and reasonable [person] would not do." Also, a standard that embodies a socially acceptable level of knowledge, experience, skill, and intelligence below which we cannot fall except at our peril.

Recklessness.   The conscious and willful disregard for what is safe based on the circumstances.

Reliance.   Basing decisions and actions on the representations of another to your detriment.

***Res ipsa loquitur* [Latin for "the thing speaks for itself"].** A term used in certain limited types of cases when the circumstances surrounding an accident constitute sufficient evidence of a defendant's negligence to support such a finding by the jury.

The following are criteria that must be met for *Res Ipsa*:

- It is common knowledge among laymen that the accident is the sort that does not ordinarily occur in the absence of negligence
- The injury producing instrumentality or conduct must have been, at some significant time, within the control of the defendant
- It must not be an injury that the plaintiff (patient) voluntarily assumed
- The evidence is more accessible to the defendant rather than to the plaintiff

The following are some examples of *Res Ipsa* cases:

- Sponge or other surgical instrument left in the patient after operation

- Operating on the wrong patient or removing the wrong organ or limb
- Death under anesthesia while undergoing a dental procedure

Respondent.   A person or party who responds as defendant in a civil suit, divorce proceeding, juvenile court, or other proceeding.

Respondeat superior **[Latin for "let the master answer"].** This doctrine means that a master is liable in certain cases for the wrongful acts of his servant, and a principal is liable for those of his agent.

Service of process.   The delivery of notice of court proceedings to the defendant.

Settlement.   Resolving a dispute before the final decision of a judge or jury.

Scope of practice.   A boundary on the types of work a professional should do. A physician's scope of practice should be limited to those tasks for which he or she is adequately prepared. This preparation is achieved through education and training.

Standard of care.   To do what a reasonable physician would do with the same or similar patient under the same or similar circumstances. The level of care a reasonable person would use in similar circumstances. The standard of care is the standard of behavior upon which the theory of negligence is based.

Statute of limitations.   A legal deadline by which a plaintiff must start a lawsuit. Also, the period during which someone can be held liable for an action or a debt.

Stipulation.   An agreement by the attorneys or parties on opposite sides of a case regarding any matter in the trial proceedings.

Strict liability.   The legal principle that a person or company who sells a product in a defective condition that is unreasonably dangerous to the ordinary user may be liable for any resulting property damage or physical injuries. Under this doctrine, liability for injury is imposed for reasons other than fault. Strict liability applies whether or not negligence or malice was involved, as long as the product was being used as was intended.

Summary judgment.   A court decision made prior to trial based upon a claim made by a party that even if the factual assertions of the opposing party are found true, they still have no legal remedies.

Subpoena.   A document issued by the authority of the court to compel a witness to appear and give testimony or produce documentary evidence in a proceeding. Failure to appear or produce evidence when requested is punishable by contempt of court.

***Subpoena Duces Tecum* [Latin for "Under penalty you shall take it with you"].**   A command by a court to a witness to produce documents. A writ or process of the same kind as the *subpoena ad testificandum*, that includes a clause requiring the witness to bring with him and produce to the court, books, papers, etc., in his hands to help elucidate the matter in issue.

Superseding intervening force.   An independent intervening force may break the connection between a wrongful act and an injury to another. If so, it acts as a superseding cause—that is, the intervening force or event sets aside, or replaces, the original wrongful act as the cause of the injury. A superseding intervening force breaks the connection between the breach of the duty of care and the injury or damage. Taking a defensive action (such as swerving to avoid an oncoming car) does not break the connection, nor does someone else's attempt to rescue the injured party.

Testify.   To give evidence as a witness in a trial, deposition, or other legal proceeding.

Testimony.   Statements made under oath.

Tort.   A breach of a duty that results in an injury for which there is a remedy at law.

Tort-feasor (also tortfeasor).   The name given to a person or persons who have committed a tort.

Unintentional tort.   A tort or wrong perpetrated by one who does not intend to do that which the law has declared wrong.

Verdict.   The decision reached by a jury or judge in a trial.

Vicarious liability.   Responsibility for the acts of a subordinate in the workplace. When a person is held responsible for the tort of another, even though the person that is being held responsible may not have done anything wrong. This is often the case with employers who are held vicariously liable for the damages caused by their employees.

Voir Dire.   The process by which attorneys and/or judges examine potential jurors to see if they are competent to sit on a jury. Having a conflict of interest with one of the parties to a lawsuit, for example, would preclude you from sitting on the jury for that litigation.

Wanton.   Grossly negligent or reckless.

Writ.   A special, written court order directing a person to perform, or refrain from performing, a specific act.

Medical Abbreviations

While there is a generalized movement in the medical community toward computerized medical charts and to the utilization of voice activated electronic dictation, most medical charts are still handwritten by physicians and nurses. The repetitive nature of the notes and the need to complete the notes quickly lead the authors to use abbreviations. While some abbreviations are standardized (e.g., SOB and CPR) and are used universally by physicians and nurses, others are unique to a specialty, geographical region, clinical setting, or single physician. Centers for Medicare and Medicaid Services allows the use of abbreviations in medical charts as long as they are consistent throughout the chart.

While abbreviations can convey a lot of specific information in a small space, they can also be ambiguous. Some abbreviations have multiple meanings. For example, "AF" can indicate adult female, amniotic fluid, atrial fibrillation, or atrial flutter. Further, abbreviations are easier to misread; that is, it is easier to decipher a full word that is written illegibly than it is an abbreviation. Some meanings of unfamiliar or ambiguous abbreviations can be gleaned from the context of the note. For example, when finding the "AD" abbreviation in a physical examination, it may be easy to tell the difference between the meanings of adult female and amniotic fluid. The meanings of others are not so easily gleaned (e.g., "PE" could stand for pulmonary edema or pulmonary embolism in a report about a chest X-ray). Because of these issues and despite their wide usage, abbreviations are discouraged by many in the academic medical community, as well as hospital risk managers and the legal defense bar. Finally, the Institute of Medicine has recently recognized misread medical abbreviations as a very common cause of medical error and has suggested the elimination of medical abbreviations as a top priority for patient safety.

The following list of common medical abbreviations should help reviewers to interpret their meaning in the charts. This list, while extensive, is not exhaustive. Therefore, clarification should be sought from the author of the note when possible.

Abbreviation	Meaning(s)
	A
A&E	Active and Equal
A&O	Alert and Oriented
A&O × 3	Alert and Oriented to Person, Place, and Time
A&P	Auscultation and Percussion, Assessment and Plan
A&W	Alive and Well
AA	Ascending Aorta
AAA	Abdominal Aortic Aneurysm
AADSI	Automobile Accident Driver-Side Impact
AAFE	Automobile Accident, Front End
AAL	Anterior Axillary Line
AAPSI	Automobile Accident Passenger-Side Impact
AAR	Antigen-Antibody Reaction, Acute Articular Rheumatism
AARE	Automobile Accident, Rear End
AAROM	Active Assisted Range of Motion
AAS	Aortic Arch Syndrome, Anthrax Anti-serum, Alcohol Abstinence Syndrome
AASP	Acute Atrophic Spinal Paralysis
Ab	Antibody, Abortion
ABA	Allergic Bronchopulmonary Aspergillosis, Arrest Before Arrival
ABD	Abdomen
ABE	Acute Bacterial Endocarditis
ABG	Arterial Blood Gas
ABM	Acute Bacterial Meningitis
ABP	Arterial Blood Pressure
AC	Acromioclavicular (Joint), Air Conduction, *Ante Cenam* (before meals)
ACD	Anemia of Chronic Disease, Allergic Contact Dermatitis
ACE	Angiotensin Converting Enzyme
ACEI	Angiotensin Converting Enzyme Inhibitor
ACI	Acute Cardiac Insufficiency
ACJ	Acromioclavicular Joint
ACL	Anterior Clavicular Line, Anterior Cruciate Ligament, Anticardiolipin (Antibody)

ACLS	Advanced Cardiac Life Support
ACM	Acetaminophen, Acute Cerebrospinal Meningitis
ACNP	Acute Care Nurse Practitioner
ACO	Alert, Cooperative, Oriented
ACS	Acute Confusional State
ACT	Activated Clotting Time
ACTH	Adrenocorticotrophic Hormone
ACTZ	Acetazolamide
AD	Alzheimer's Dementia, Admitting Diagnosis, *Auris Dexter* (right ear)
Ad lib	As Needed, As Desired
ADA	Anterior Descending Artery
ADC	AIDS Demential Complex
ADD	Attention Deficit Disorder
Adeno Ca	Adenocarcinoma
ADH	Antidiuretic Hormone (vasopressin)
ADHD	Attention Deficit Hyperactivity Disorder
ADJ	Adjuvant Chemotherapy
ADL	Activities of Daily Living
ADM	Administered, Administration
ADV	Advised
AED	Automated External Defibrillator
AEH	Atypical Endometrial Hyperplasia
AF	Adult Female, Amniotic Fluid, Atrial Fibrillation, Atrial Flutter, Afebrile
AFB	Acid Fast Bacillus
A-fib	Atrial Fibrillation
AFL	Atrial Flutter
AGTT	Abnormal Glucose Tolerance Test
AH	Abdominal Hysterectomy
AHD	Acute Heart Disease, Autoimmune Hemolytic Disease
AHF	Acute Heart Failure
AHJ	Artificial Hip Joint
AHP	Acute Hemorrhagic Pancreatitis
AI	Aortic Insufficiency, Artificial Intelligence
AICD	Automated Internal Cardiac Defibrillator, Automated Implantable Cardiac Defibrillator
AIS	Adenocarcinoma in Situ
AK	Above the Knee

AKA	Above the Knee Amputation, Also Known As
ALBP	Acute Low Back Pain
ALL	Acute Lymphocytic Leukemia
ALS	Acute Lumbar Strain, Advanced Life Support, Amyotrophic Lateral Sclerosis
ALVF	Acute Left Ventricular Failure
AM	Anteromedial
AMA	Against Medical Advice
AMB	Ambulate, Ambulatory
AMI	Acute Myocardial Infarction
AML	Acute Myelogenous Leukemia
ANA	Antinuclear Antibody
ANB	Aspiration Needle Biopsy
ANP	Atrial Natruretic Peptide, Advanced Nurse Practitioner
Ant	Anterior
Anx	Anxiety
Ao	Aorta
AOB	Alcohol on Breath
AODM	Adult Onset Diabetes Mellitus
AOE	Acute Otitis Externa
AOM	Acute Otitis Media
AP	Angina Pectoris, Anterior-Posterior, Apical Pulse, Appendectomy, Arterial Pressure, Aspiration Pneumonia
APAP	Acetaminophen (paracetamol)
APC	Atrial Premature Contraction; Acetylsalicylic Acid, Phenacetin, and Caffeine (antipyretic)
APR	Anteroposterior Resection
ARB	Angiotensin Receptor Blocker
ARC	AIDS-Related Complex
ARDS	Adult Respiratory Distress Syndrome
ARF	Acute Renal Failure, Acute Respiratory Failure
AROM	Active Range of Motion, Artificial Rupture of Membranes
AS	Auris Sinistrae (left ear), Aortic Stenosis, Asystole
ASA	Acetylsalicylic Acid (aspirin)
ASAP	As Soon as Possible
ASC	Ascending
ASD	Atrial Septal Defect

ASH	Asymmetrical Septal Hypertrophy
ASIS	Anterior Superior Iliac Spine
ASU	Ambulatory Surgery Unit
AT	Anterior Tibial, Achilles Tendon
ATLS	Advanced Trauma Life Support
ATN	Acute Tubular Necrosis
ATP	Attending Physician, Autoimmune Thrombocytopenic Purpura
ATR	Achilles Tendon Reflex
AU	*Auris Unitas* (both ears), *Ad Usum* (according to custom), *Aurum* (Gold)
AUB	Abnormal Uterine Bleeding
AUSC	Auscultation
AV	Atrioventricular, Acne Vulgaris, Arteriovenous, Aortic Valve
AVHD	Acquired Valvular Heart Disease
AVI	Aortic Valve Insufficiency
AVM	Arteriovenous Malformations
AVN	Atrioventricular Node, Avascular Necrosis
AVR	Aortic Valve Replacement, Aortic Valve Regurgitation
AVS	Aortic Valve Stenosis
AX	Axial, Axillary
AXL	Axillary Line
AZT	Azidothymidine (zidovudine)

B

B&C	Biopsy and Curettage
BA	Barium, Blood Alcohol
Bab +	Babinski Reflex (Positive)
BAC	Blood Alcohol Concentration
BAL	Bronchoalveolar Lavage, Blood Alcohol Level
BASO	Basophil (leukocytes)
BAT	Basic Aid Training, Blunt Abdominal Trauma
BB	Bed Bath, Breakthrough Bleeding, Blood Bank
BBA	Born Before Arrival, Extramural Birth
BBB	Blood Brain Barrier, Bundle Branch Block
BBBB	Bilateral Bundle Branch Block
BBT	Basal Body Temperature

BC	Birth Control, Blood Culture, Breast Cancer, Bronchial Carcinoma, Bone Conduction
BC+	Blood Culture Positive
BCA	Balloon Catheter Angioplasty
BCG	Bacille Calmette-Guérin, Bacillus Calmette-Guérin Vaccine
BCNU	Carmustine
BCP	Birth Control Pill
BCT	Blunt Chest Trauma
BE	Barium Enema
BF	Black Female
BHCG	Beta Human Chorionic Gonadotropin (pregnancy test)
BHT	Blunt Head Trauma
BIBA	Brought in by Ambulance
BIBF	Brought in by Family (friend)
BID	Two Times a Day
Bilat	Bilateral
BK	Below the Knee
BKA	Below-the-Knee Amputation
BL	Blood Loss
BLE	Both Lower Extremities
BLS	Basic Life Support
BM	Black Male, Bowel Movement
BMI	Body Mass Index
BNP	Brain Natruretic Peptide
BOOP	Bronchiolitis Obliterans with Organizing Pneumonia
BPD	Bipolar Disease
BPH	Benign Prostatic Hypertrophy
BRADY	Bradycardia
BRBPR	Bright Red Blood Per Rectum
Bronch	Bronchoscopy, Bronchoscope
BS	Bowel Sounds, Blood Sugar
BSA	Body Surface Area
BT	Bleeding Time
BUN	Blood Urea Nitrogen
BW	Birth Weight
BX	Biopsy

C

C diff	Clostridium Difficle
C sect, C-section	Cesarean Section
C&C	Cold and Clammy
C&M	Cocaine and Morphine
C&S	Culture and Sensitivity
C/C/E	Cyanosis, Clubbing, Edema
C/M	Counts Per Minute
C/O	Care of, Complains of
C/S	Cesarean Section
C1, C2, C3 ...	Cervical Vertebrae 1, 2, 3 ...
CA	Cancer, Carcinoma
CAB	Coronary Artery Bypass
CABG	Coronary Artery Bypass Graft
CAD	Coronary Artery Disease
CAE	Carotid Artery Endarterectomy
CAF	Chronic Atrial Fibrillation
CAH	Chronic Active Hepatitis
CAP	Community Acquired Pneumonia
CAPD	Continuous Ambulatory Peritoneal Dialysis
CAT	Computer Axial Tomography
CBC	Complete Blood Count
CBE	Chronic Bacterial Endocarditis
CBF	Cerebral Blood Flow, Coronary Blood Flow
CC	Chief Complaint, Cubic Centimeter
CCA	Circumflex Coronary Artery, Common Carotid Artery
CCE	Cyanosis, Clubbing or Edema
CCMSU	Clean Catch Midstream Urine
CCPD	Continuous Cycling Peritoneal Dialysis
CCRC	Continuous Care Retirement Community
CCU	Cardiac Care Unit
CD	Cadaver Donor, Cavaderic Donor, Crohn's Disease
CDH	Congenital Dislocation of the Hip, Congenital Dysplasia of Hip
CEZ	Cefazolin
CF	Cystic Fibrosis
CHD	Congenital Hip Dislocation, Congenital Heart Disease
CHF	Congestive Heart Failure

CHI	Closed Head Injury
CHT	Closed Head Trauma
CI	Cardiac Insufficiency, Cerebral Infarction, Cognitive Impairment
CIRC	Circulation, Circumference, Circumcision
CIS	Carcinoma in Situ
CJD	Cholecysto-Jejuno-Duodenostomy, Creutzfeld-Jacob Disease
CKS	Classic Kaposi Sarcoma
CLBBB	Complete Left Bundle Branch Block
CLBP	Chronic Low Back Pain
CLD	Chronic Liver Disease, Chronic Lung Disease
CLE	Continuous Lumbar Epidural (anesthesia).
CLL	Chronic Lymphocytic Leukemia
CM	Congenital Malformation, Congestive Myocardiopathy, Continuous Murmur, Contrast Medium, Costal Margin
cm^2	Square Centimeter
cm^3	Cubic Centimeter
CMD	Chronic Maintenance Dialysis
CMF	Cyclophosphamide, Methotrexate, and 5-Fluorouracil, Cytoxan, Methotrexate and 5-Fluorouracil
CMF/VP	Cyclophosphamide, Methotrexate, 5-Fluorouracil, Vincristine, and Prednisone
CML	Chronic Myelogenous Leukemia
CMS	Centers for Medicare and Medicaid Services
CMV	Cytomegalovirus
CN II–XII	Cranial Nerves Two Through Twelve
CNS	Central Nervous System
CO	Cardiac Output, Carbon Monoxide
CO_2	Carbon Dioxide
COA	Condition on Admission
COD	Cause of Death, Condition on Discharge
COLD	Chronic Obstructive Lung Disease
COPD	Chronic Obstructive Pulmonary Disease
CORF	Comprehensive Outpatient Rehabilitation Facility
COX–II	Cyclooxygenase-II
CP	Cerebral Palsy, Chest Pain
CPAP	Continuous Positive Airway Pressure

CPD	Cephalopelvic Disproportion, Chronic Peritoneal Dialysis
CPK	Creatinine Phosphokinase
CPOE	Computerized Pharmacy Order Entry
CPR	Cardiopulmonary Resuscitation
CREST	Calcinosis, Raynaud phenomenon, Esophageal motility disorders, Sclerodactyly, and Telangiectasia
CRF	Chronic Renal Failure
CRL	Crown-Rump Length
CRNA	Certified Registered Nurse Anesthetist
CS	Cesarean Section
C-spine	Cervical Spine
CT	Chest Tube, Computerized Axial Tomography, Cardiothoracic, Cadaric Transplant
CTO	Cervicothoracic Orthosis
CTS	Carpal Tunnel Syndrome
CV	Cardiovascular
CVA	Cerebrovascular Accident
CVHD	Congenital Valvular Heart Disease
CVP	Central Venous Pressure
CXR	Chest X-ray
C-x-ray	Chest X-ray

D

D&C	Dilatation and Curettage
D&E	Dilatation and Evacuation, Dilatation and Extraction
D/A	Date of Accident, Date of Admission
D/DW	Dextrose in Distilled Water
D/H	Drug History
D/NS	Dextrose in Normal Saline
D/W	Dextrose in Water, Discussed With
D10NS	Dextrose in 10% Normal Saline
D1OW	10% Aqueous Dextrose Solution
D50	Dextrose 50% solution
D51 $\frac{1}{2}$ NS	5% Dextrose in $\frac{1}{2}$ Normal Saline
D5NS	Dextrose 5% Normal Saline
D5RL	Dextrose 5% Ringer's Lactate
D5W	5% Dextrose in Water

DA	Descending Aorta, Developmental Age
DALYs	Disability-Adjusted Life Years
DAT	Dementia of the Alzheimer's Type, Diet as Tolerated
Db	Decibel
DB	Disability
dB	Decibel
DBP	Diastolic Blood Pressure
DC	Discharge, Discontinue
DC&B	Dilation, Curettage and Biopsy
DC'd	Discontinued
DCIS	Ductal Carcinoma In Situ (type of breast cancer)
DCM	Dilated Cardiomyopathy
DD	Discharge Diagnosis, Dry Dressing
DDAVP	Desmopressin Acetate, Desmopressin Test for Urine Osmolality
Ddx	Differential Diagnosis
DES	Diethylstilbestrol
DEXA	Dual-Energy X-ray Absorptiometry
DFI	Disease-Free Interval
DHE	Dihydroergotamine
DHEA	Dehydroepiandrosterone
DI	Date of Injury, Diabetes Insipidus
Diag	Diagnosis, Diagnostic
DIC	Disseminated Intravascular Coagulation
DIS	Dispense
DISH	Diffuse Idiopathic Skeletal Hyperostosis
DISL	Dislocate; Dislocation
DISP	Disposition
DIST	Distal, Distended
DIW	Dextrose in Water
DJD	Degenerative Joint Disease
DKA	Diabetic Ketoacidosis, Did Not Keep Appointment
DLS	Date Last Seen
DM	Diabetes Mellitus, Diastolic Murmur
DME	Durable Medical Equipment
DNA	Did Not Attend (clinic), Deoxyriboneucleic Acid
DND	Died a Natural Death
DNI	Do Not Intubate
DNI/DNR	Do Not Intubate, Do Not Resuscitate

DNKA	Did Not Keep Appointment
DNR	Do Not Resuscitate, Dorsal Nerve Root
DNS	Did Not Show for Appointment
DO	Doctor of Osteopathy, Doctor of Osteopathic Medicine, Doctor of Ophthalmology, Doctor of Optometry, Oxygen Diffusion, Dorsal Outflow
DOA	Day of Admission, Dead on Arrival
DOB	Date of Birth
DOC	Died of Other Causes
DOD	Date of Death
DOE	Date of Examination, Dyspnea on Exertion
DOES	Disorder of Excessive Somnolence (narcolepsy)
DOI	Date of Injury
DPC	Direct Patient Care, Delayed Primary Closure, Diffuse Pulmonary Disease
DPH	Diphenylhydantoin
DPL	Diagnostic Peritoneal Lavage
DPM	Doctor of Podiatric Medicine
DPT	Diphtheria, Pertussis, Tetanus
DR	Delivery Room, Diabetic Retinopathy, Diagnostic Radiology, Dorsal Root, Dressing
dr	Dram
DRE	Digital Rectal Examination
Drng	Drainage
Drsg	Dressing
DS	Right Eye
DSA	Digital Substraction Angiography
DSD	Dry Sterile Dressing
DSG	Dry Sterile Gauze
DSV	Digital Subtraction Venacavography, Digital Subtraction Venography
DT	Delirium Tremens
DTP	Diphtheria and Tetanus Toxoids with Pertussis (killed, whole organism)
DTR	Deep Tendon Reflexes
DTZ	Diltiazem
DU	Diagnosis Undetermined, Duodenal Ulcer, Duplex Ultrasound
DUB	Dysfunctional Uterine Bleeding
DUD	Duodenal Ulcer Disease

DVT	Deep Venous Thrombosis
Dx	Diagnosis
DX	Dextran, Dicloxacillin, Discharged, Disease, Diagnosis
DXA	Dual-Energy X-ray Absorptiometry
DXD	Discontinued
DXM	Dexamethasone, Dextromethorphan

E

EA	Epidural Anesthesia
EBL	Estimated Blood Loss
EBV	Epstein-Barr Virus
Echo	Echocardiogram
ECMO	Extracorporeal Membrane Oxygenation
ECP	External Counter Pulsation
ECR	Extracorporeal Circulation
ED	Emergency Department
EDC	Estimated Date of Confinement
EECP	Enhanced External Counter Pulsation
EEG	Electroencephalogram
EENT	Ears, Eyes, Nose, and Throat
EF	Ejection Fraction
EKG	Electrocardiogram
EMG	Electromyogram
EMT	Emergency Medical Technicians
Endo	Endoscopy, Endoscope
ENT	Ears, Nose, and Throat
EOM	Extraocular Movement
EOMI	Extraocular Motions Intact
EP	Ectopic Pregnancy
EPS	Electophysiologic Study
ER	Emergency Room
ERCP	Endoscopic Retrograde Cholangiopancreatography
ESR	Erythrocyte Sedimentation Rate
ESRF	End Stage Renal Failure
ESWL	Extracorporeal Shockwave Lithotripsy
ET	Endotracheal
ETOH	Ethanol (alcohol)
ETT	Endotracheal Tube
EXT	Extremity

F

F/U	Follow Up
FACC	Fellow of the American College of Cardiology
FACOG	Fellow of the American College of Obstetrics and Gynecology
FACP	Fellow of the American College of Physicians
FACS	Fellow of the American College of Surgeons
FB	Foreign Body, Fingerbreadth
FBS	Fasting Blood Sugar
FCA	Fracture, Complete, Angulated
FCC	Fracture, Complete, Comminuted; Fracture, Compound, Comminuted
FCCC	Fracture, Complete, Comminuted, Compound
Fe	Iron
Fe SO$_4$	Ferrous Sulfate
FEF	Forced Expiratory Flow
FEKG	Fetal Electrocardiogram
FEV	Forced Expiratory Volume
FH	Family History
FHT	Fetal Heart Tones
FiO$_2$	Fraction of Inspired Oxygen
FLAIR	Fluid-Attenuated Inversion Recovery (an MRI technique)
FMF	Familial Mediterranean Fever
FNP	Family Nurse Practitioner
FO	Fecal Output
FOBT	Fecal Occult Blood Testing
FROM	Full Range of Motion
FSC	Fracture, Simple Comminuted
FTKA	Failed to Keep Appointment
FTND	Full Term Normal Delivery
FU	Follow Up
FUO	Fever of Unknown Origin
FVC	Forced Vital Capacity
FWB	Full Weight Bearing
Fx	Fracture

G

G	Gravida, Glycine, Gram, Histopathological Grading
G −	Gram Negative

G +	Gram Positive
G/M	Granulocyte/Macrophage
g/ml	Grams Per Milliliter
G/P	Gravida/Para
GA	General Anesthetic/Anesthesia, Gestational Age
GB	Gallbladder
GBD	Gallbladder Disease
GBS	Guillain-Barré Syndrome, Group B Streptococcus
GCA	Giant Cell Arteritis
GCS	Glasgow Coma Scale
G-CSF	Granulocyte Colony Stimulating Factor Promotes Production of White Blood Cells
GE	Gastroenteritis, Gastroesophageal
GERD	Gastroesophageal Reflux Disease
GES	Gastroesophageal Sphincter
GF	Greenfield Filter
GFR	Glomerular Filtration Rate
GG	Gamma Globulin
GGT	Gamma-Glutamyltransferase
GH	General Health
GHT	Growth Hormone Therapy
gluc	Glucose
gm. Neg	Gram Negative
GMC	General Medical Clinic
GMR	Gallops, Murmurs, Rubs
GN	Gram-Negative, Graduate Nurse
GNC	General Nursing Care, Geriatric Nurse Clinician, Gram-Negative Cocci
GND	Gram-Negative Diplococci
GNID	Gram-Negative Intracellular Diplococci
GNP	Gerontologic Nurse Practitioner, Geriatric Nurse Practitioner
GNR	Gram-Negative Rods
GP	Gram Positive
GPC	Gram-Positive Cocci
GPR	Gram-Positive Rods
GRAV	Gravida (a pregnant woman)
GSW	Gun Shot Wound
GT	Gait Training
gt, gtt	Drop, Drops

GTT	Glucose Tolerance Test
Gtts	Drops Per Minute
GU	Genitourinary, Gastric Ulcer, Gonococcal Urethritis
GUD	Gastric Ulcer Disease
GvHD	Graft Versus Host Disease
GVHR	Graft Versus Host Reaction

H

H&E	Hemorrhages and Exudates
H&P	History and Physical Examination
h.s.	At the Hour of Sleep
h/o	History Of
H_2O	Water
H_2O_2	Hydrogen Peroxide
HAA	Hepatitis-Associated Antigen
HAP	Hospital-Acquired Pneumonia
HCG	Human Chorionic Gonadotropin
HCL	Hairy Cell Leukemia
HCl	Hydrochloric Acid, Hydrochloride
HCM	Hypertrophic Cardiomyopathy
HCO_3	Bicarbonate
HCT, Hct, hct	Hematocrit, Helical-Computed Tomography, Hydrochlorothiazide
HCTZ	Hydrochlorothiazide
HDC	High-Dose Chemotherapy
HDCT	High-Dose Chemotherapy
HDCT/SCR	High-Dose Chemotherapy with Stem Cell Rescue
HDCT/SCT	High-Dose Chemotherapy with Stem Cell Transplant
HDL	High-Density Lipoprotein
HEENT	Head, Eyes, Ears, Nose, and Throat
Hep A	Hepatitis, Type A
Hep B	Hepatitis, Type B
Hep C	Hepatitis, Type C
HHA	Home Health Aide, Home Health Agency, Hand-Held Assistance
HHV	Human Herpes Virus
HIDA	Hepatic Iminodiacetic Acid (imaging or scanning)
HIT	Heparin-Induced Thrombocytopenia
HIV	Human Immunodeficiency Virus

HIV/AIDS	Human Immunodeficiency Virus/Acquired Immune Deficiency Syndrome
H-J	Hepato-Jugular
HJR	Hepato-Jugular Reflux
HO	History of, House Officer
HP	Hemipelvectomy, Hot Pack
HPI	History of Present Illness
HPV	Human Papilloma Virus
HQoL	Health-Related Quality of Life
HR	Heart Rate, High Risk, Hospital Record, Hour
HRT	Hormone Replacement Therapy
HSV	Herpes Simplex Virus
HT	Heart, Height, Hospital Treatment, Hypertension, Hyperthyroidism
HTN	Hypertension
HV	Hepatic Vein, Herpes Virus, Home Visit, Hospital Visit, Hyperventilation
Hx	History
HZV	Herpes Zoster Virus

I

IA	Iliac Artery
IAN	Intern Admission Note
IBD	Inflammatory Bowel Disease
ICE	Ice, Compression, Elevation
ICH	Intracerebral Hemorrhage
ICP	Intracerebral Pressure
ICU	Intensive Care Unit
IDDM	Insulin-Dependent Diabetes Mellitus
IM	Intramuscular
IMP	Impression
IOP	Intraocular Pressure
IPPB	Intermittent Positive Pressure Breathing
IS	Intercostal Space
ITP	Idiopathic Thrombocytopenic Purpura
IUD	Intrauterine Device
IV	Intravenous
IVC	Inferior Vena Cava
IVCA	Intravenous Contrast Agent
IVCM	Intravenous Contrast Medium

IVDA	Intravenous Drug Addict (abuser)
IVDU	Intravenous Drug User
IVF	In Vitro Fertilization, Intravascular Filter
IVP	Intravenous Pyelogram
IVSD	Interventricular Septal Defect, Intraventricular Septal Defect

J

JCD	Jakob-Creutzfeldt Disease
JD	Juvenile Diabetes
JODM	Juvenile-Onset Diabetes Mellitus
JP	Jackson-Pratt
JPD	Jackson-Pratt Drain
JRA	Juvenile Rheumatoid Arthritis
JT	Joint
JUV	Juvenile
JV	Jugular Vein, Jugulovenous
JVD	Jugular Venous Distention
JVP	Jugulovenous Pulse, Jugulovenous Pressure

K

K	Potassium
KA	Ketoacidosis
kCal	Kilogram Calorie, Kilocalorie
KCL	Potassium Chloride
KI	Potassium Iodide
KLS	Kidney, Liver, and Spleen
KO	Keep Open
KOH	Potassium Hydroxide
KS	Kaposi's Sarcoma
KUB	Kidneys, Ureters, and Bladder
KVO	Keep Vein Open
K-wire	Kirschner Wire

L

L&A	Light and Accommodation
L&D	Labor and Delivery
L&W	Living and Well
L1, L2, L3 ...	Lumbar Vertebra 1, 2, 3 ...
LAC	Lactate, Laceration

LAD	Left Anterior Descending Artery
LB	Pound
LBBB	Left Bundle Branch Block
LBP	Lower Back Pain
LBPS	Low Back Pain Syndrome
LCM	Left Costal Margin
LCTA	Lungs Clear to Auscultation
LCTAP	Lungs Clear to Auscultation and Percussion
LDL	Low-Density Lipoprotein
LES	Lower-Esophageal Sphincter
LF	Lung Fields
LFC	Lung Fields Clear
LFTs	Liver Function Tests
LGIH	Lower-Gastrointestinal Hemorrhage
LGV	Lymphogranuloma Venereum
LLE	Left Lower Extremity
LLL	Left Lower Lobe
LLLF	Left Lower Lung Field
LLQ	Left Lower Quadrant
LMA	Left Main Artery
LMD	Left Midline Deviation
LMP	Last Menstrual Period
LMWH	Low Molecular Weight Heparin
LN	Lymph Node
LOA	Left Occipitoanterior
LOC	Loss of Consciousness
LOP	Left Occipitoposterior
LOS	Length of Stay
LOT	Left Occiput Transverse
LP	Lumbar Puncture
LPN	Licensed Practical Nurse
LQTS	Long Quadrant Syndrome
LRQ	Lower Right Quadrant
LS	Lumbosacral
LS spine	Lumbosacral Spine
LSK	Liver, Spleen, and Kidney
LT	Left
LTC	Long-Term Care
LTCF	Long-Term Care Facility
LTD	Limited

LUE	Left Upper Extremity
LUL	Left Upper Lobe
LULF	Left Upper Lung Field
LUQ	Left Upper Quadrant
LV	Left Ventricle
LVEP	Left Ventricular End Diastolic Pressure
LVH	Left Ventricular Hypertrophy
LYMPH	Lymphocyte

M

M	Male, Meter
MAB	Monoclonal Antibodies
MAC	Mycobacterium Avium Complex
MACE	Major Adverse Cardiac Event
MBC	Maximum Breathing Capacity
MCG	Microgram
MCL	Midclavicular Line
MCV	Mean Corpuscular Volume
MD	Muscular Dystrophy, Medical Doctor, Macular Degeneration, Maintenance Dialysis, Major Depression, Manic Depression, Mitral Disease, Moderate Disability
MDA	Medical Doctor Aware (i.e., the nurse has notified the physician in charge of the situation)
Meds	Medication
MEQ	Milliequivalents
MEQ/L	Milliequivalents Per Liter
METS	Metastasis
MG	Milligram, Magnesium
MGSO$_4$	Magnesium Sulfate
MH	Medication History, Mental Health
MI	Myocardial Infarction, Mitral Insufficiency
MIC	Maximum Inhibitory Concentration
ML	Milliliter
Mm	Millimeter
Mm/hg	Millimeters of Mercury
MMPI	Minnesota Multiphasic Personality Inventory (test)
MMR	Measles, Mumps, and Rubella Vaccine
MOM	Milk of Magnesia
MONO	Monocyte, Mononeucleosis

MONO SPOT	Test for Mononucleosis
MRA	Magnetic Resonance Angiography
MRI	Magnetic Resonance Imaging
MRSA	Methacillin-Resistant Staph Aureus
MS	Motor Strength, Morphine Sulfate, Multiple Sclerosis, Mitral Stenosis, Myasthenic Syndrome (Lambert-Eaton syndrome)
MSL	Midsternal Line
MSSA	Methacillin Sensitive Staph Aureus
MSU	Midstream Urine, Medicine-Surgery Unit
MTD	Right Eardrum
MTS	Left Eardrum
MTX	Methotrexate
MUGA	Multiple-Gated Acquisition Scan
Multip	Multiparous (many births)
MV	Mitral Valve
MVA	Motor Vehicle Accident
MVP	Mitral Valve Prolapse
MVR	Mitral Valve Regurgitation, Mitral Valve Replacement
MVS	Mistral Valve Stenosis
MVV	Maximum Voluntary Ventilation
Myop	Myopia

N

N	Nitrogen
N&V	Nausea and Vomiting
NA	Sodium
NACL	Sodium Chloride
NAD	No Acute Distress
NAD	No Appreciable Disease, Nothing Abnormal Detected
NB	New Born, Note Well
NBS	Normal Breath Sounds, Normal Bowel Sounds
NC/AT	Normocephalic / Atraumatic
NCA	Nodulocystic Acne
NCS	Nerve Conduction Study
NED	No Evidence of Disease
NEG	Negative
NER	No Evidence of Reoccurrence

NERD	No Evidence of Recurrent Disease
NG	Nasogastric
NGA	No Gross Abnormality
NGT	Nasogastric Tube
NGU	Non-Gonnacoccal Urethritis
NH	Nursing Home, Neurological History
NICU	Neurologic Intensive Care Unit, Neurosurgical Intensive Care Unit
NIDDM	Non-Insulin-Dependent Diabetes Mellitus
NKA	No Known Allergies
NKDA	No Known Drug Allergies
NMR	Nuclear Magnetic Resonance
Non rep	Do Not Repeat
Non-STEMI	Non-ST Wave Elevation Myocardial Infarction
NOS	Not Otherwise Specified
NP	Nurse Practitioner
NPH	Normal Pressure Hydrocephalus, Neutral Protein Hagadorn, Nucleus Palpulpus Herniation, Nasopharngeal, Nasopharynx, Neonatal Primary Hyperparathyroidism
NPO	Nothing by Mouth
NQMI	Non-Q Wave Myocardial Infraction
NS	Normal Saline
NSAID	Nonsteroidal Anti-Inflammatory Drug
NSR	Normal Sinus Rhythm
NSVD	Normal Spontaneous Vaginal Delivery
NTMI	Nontransmural Myocardial Infarction
NTNG	Nontoxic Nodular Goiter
NTP	Normal Temperature and Pressure
NUG	Necrotizing Ulcerative Gingivitis
NVD	Normal Vaginal Delivery; Nausea, Vomiting, and Diarrhea

O

O&E	Observation and Examination
O&P	Ova and Parasite
O.&A.	Odontectomy and Alveolectomy
O/E	On Examination
O_2	Oxygen
OA	Osteoarthritis

OB	Obstetrics
OB/GYN	Obstetrics and Gynecology
OBL	Oblique
OBP	Orthostatic Blood Pressure
OBP	Ova, Blood, and Parasites
OBS	Observer, Obstetrics, Organic Brain Syndrome (dementia)
OCD	Obsessive-Compulsive Disorder
OD	Overdose, Each Day, *Oculus Dexter* (right eye)
ODA	On Day of Admission
OGTT	Oral Glucose Tolerance Test
OMA	Obtuse Marginal Artery
OMS	Organic Mental Syndrome (dementia)
ONC	Oncology
OOB	Out of Bed
OOBTC	Out of Bed to Chair
OPC	Outpatient Clinic
OPT	Outpatient Treatment, Outpatient
OPV	Oral Polio Vaccine
OR	Operating Room
ORIF	Open Reduction Internal Fixation
Ortho, ORTH	Orthopedics
OS	*Oculus Sinistrae* (left eye)
OSAS	Obstructive Sleep Apnea Syndrome
OT	Objective Test, Occupational Therapy
OTC	Over the Counter (A medication that can be obtained without a prescription)
OU	*Oculus Uterque* (each eye)
OV	Office Visit
Ox	Oxygen

P

P&D	Prepped and Draped
PA	Physician Assistant
PAC	Premature Atrial Contraction
PAD	Peripheral Arterial Disease, Peripheral Arteriosclerotic Disease
PADP	Pulmonary Artery Diastolic Pressure
PAEDP	Pulmonary Artery End-Diastolic Pressure
PAL	Posterior Axillary Line

PALS	Pediatric Advanced Life Support
PAP	Pulmonary Artery Pressure
PAP	Papanicolaou Smear or Test
Para I, II, III	Number of Pregnancies, 1, 2, 3 …
Path	Pathology
PBO	Placebo
pc	*Post Cenam* (after meals), Posterior Cervical, Present Complaint
PC	After Meals
PCA	Patient-Controlled Analgesia
PCD	Pneumatic Compression Device
PCL	Posterior Cruciate Ligament
PCN	Penicillin
PCO	Polycystic Ovaries
PCO_2	Partial Pressure of Carbon Dioxide, Pressure of Carbon Dioxide
PCOD	Polycystic Ovarian Disease
PCP	Phencyclidine, *Pneumocystis Carinii* Pneumonia, Primary Care Physician
PCR	Polymerase Chain Reaction
PCV	Packed Cell Volume
PD	Peritoneal Dialysis, Penrose Drain
PDA	Patent Ductus Arteriosus., Posterior Descending Artery
PDUSF	Prepped and Draped in the Usual Sterile Fashion
PE	Physical Examination, Pulmonary Embolism, Pre-Eclampsia, Pulmonary Edema
PEAP	Positive End-Airway Pressure
Peds	Pediatrics
PEEP	Positive End-Expiratory Pressure
PEF	Peak Expiratory Flow
PEG	Percutaneous Endoscopic Gastrotomy
PEN	Parenteral Nutrition
PER OS	By Mouth
per/os	By Mouth
PERRLA	Pupils: Equal, Round, Reactive to Light and Accommodation
PET	Positron Emission Tomography
PFO	Patent Foramen Ovale
PFT	Pulmonary Function Test

PGY − 1	Post Graduate Year One, Intern
PGY − 2	Post Graduate Year Two, Resident
PGY − 3	Post Graduate Year Three, Senior Resident
PH	Portal Hypertension, Past History
PHN	Phenacetin, Pulmonary Hypertension
PHX	Past History
PI	Present Illness
PIC	Peripherally Inserted Catheter
PID	Pelvic Inflammatory Disease
PIH	Pregnancy-Induced Hypertension
PIL	Peripheral Intravenous Line
PKU	Phenylketonuria
PL	Peritoneal Lavage
PM	Postmortem
PM&R	Physical Medicine and Rehabilitation
PMB	Postmenopausal Bleeding
PMP	Previous Menstrual Period, Past Menstrual Period
PNC	Prenatal Care
PND	Paroxysmal Nocturnal Dyspnea, Postnatal Day
PNS	Paraneoplastic Syndrome
PO	Postoperative
PO$_2$	Pressure of Oxygen
POC	Products of Conception
POD	Postoperative Day
POME	Persistent Otitis Media with Effusion
poss	Possible
post	Posterior, Postmortem
postop	Postoperative
post-op	Postoperative(Ly)
PP	Phosphoprotein Phosphatase, Positive Pressure, Postpartum, Postprandial, Presenting Problem
PPD	Packs Per Day, Permanent Partial Disability, Purified Protein Derivative (of tuberculin)
PPT	Plasma Pregnancy Test
PR	Per Rectum
PRBC	Packed Red Blood Cells
Pre-op	Prior to Operation, Before Operation
Primip	Primipara, Primiparity
PRL	Proline
PRN	When Necessary

Pro	Proline
PROM	Passive Range of Motion, Premature Rupture of Membranes
Pro-time	Prothrombin Time
PRT	Patient Refused Test
PS	Present Symptoms
PSA	Prostate-Specific Antigen
PSC	Primary Sclerosing Cholangitis
PSD	Presurgical Diagnosis, Postsurgical Diagnosis
PSGN	Post-Streptococcal Glomerulonephritis
PT	Patient, Physical Therapy, Prothrombin Time
PTA	Prior to Admission, Prior to Arrival, Percutaneous Transluminal Angioplasty, Physical Therapy Assistant, Persistent Truncus Arteriosis
PTCA	Percutaneous Transluminal Coronary Angioplasty
PTH	Parathyroid Hormone
PTT	Partial Thromboplastin Time
PTX	Pneumothorax
PUD	Peptic Ulcer Disease
PVC	Premature Ventricular Contraction
PVH	Pulmonary Vascular Hypertension
PVR	Peripheral Vascular Resistance
PVS	Persistent Vegetative State
PWB	Partial Weight Bearing
PWP	Pulmonary Wedge Pressure
PWS	Port Wine Stain (nevus flammeus)
PX	Prognosis
PZB	Tripelennamine HCL

Q

Q	Each, Every
q.d.	Every Day
q.h.	Every Hour
q.h.s.	Every Night at Bed Time
q.s.	As Much as Suffices
Q12	Every 12 Hours
Q24	Every 24 Hours
Q8	Every 8 Hours
Qh	Every Hour
Qhs	Every Night at Sleep

QID	Four Times a Day
QL	As Much as Desired
Qn	Every Night
Qod	Every Other Day
Q-TwiST	Time Without Symptoms or Toxicity
QW	Q-Wave

R

R.Ph.	Registered Pharmacist
R/G/M	Rubs, Gallops, or Murmurs
RA	Right Atrium, Rheumatoid Arthritis
RAN	Resident Admission Note
RAP	Right Atrial Pressure
RBBB	Right Bundle Branch Block
RBC	Red Blood Cell
RCA	Right Coronary Artery, Right Circumflex Artery
RCM	Right Costal Margin
RDS	Respiratory Distress Syndrome
RE	Right Eye
REM	Rapid Eye Movement
RES	Reticuloendothelial System
Retic	Reticulocyte
RF	Respiratory Failure, Rheumatoid Factor
RFA	Radiofrequency Ablation
Rh	Rh Blood Group Systems
RHC	Rural Health Clinic
RHD	Rheumatic Heart Disease
RICE	Rest, Ice, Compression, and Elevation
RIND	Reversible Ischemic Neurologic Deficit
RLE	Right Lower Extremity
RLL	Right Lower Lobe
RLLF	Right Lower Lung Field
RLQ	Right Lower Quadrant
RM	Radical Mastectomy
RMD	Right Midline Deviation
RN	Registered Nurse
RO or R/O	Rule Out
ROA	Right Occipitoanterior
ROAP	Rule Out Appendicitis
ROM	Range of Motion

ROMI	Rule Out Myocardial Infarction
ROP	Right Occipital Posterior
ROS	Removal of Sutures, Review of Systems
ROT	Right Occiput Transverse
RP	Retrograde Pyelogram
RPN	Resident Progress Note
RR	Respiratory Rate, Recovery Room
RS	Review of Symptoms
RSC	Right Subclavian
RSCV	Right Subclavian Vein
RSD	Reflex Sympathetic Dystrophy
RSDS	Reflex Sympathetic Dystrophy Syndrome
RSI	Rapid Sequence Induction, Rapid Sequence Intubation, or Repetition Strain Injury
RSR	Regular Sinus Rhythm
RSS	Rectosigmoidoscopy
RST	Right Sacrotransverse Position
RT	Rectal Temperature, Registered Technician, Renal Transplantation, Respiratory Therapist/Therapy, Response Time, Refractory Time, Radiation Therapy
RTA	Renal Tubular Acidosis
RTC	Return to Clinic, Rape Treatment Center
RTs	Respiratory Therapists
RUE	Right Upper Extremity
RUL	Right Upper Lobe
RULF	Right Upper Lung Field
RUQ	Right Upper Quadrant
RV	Residual Volume of Lung, Right Ventricle
RVH	Right Ventricular Hypertrophy
RVT	Renal Vein Thrombosis
RW	Rolling Walker
Rx	Treatment, Therapy, Prescription
c̄	Latin for "Cum" or With

S

s	*Sine* (without)
S & sx	Signs and Symptoms
s̄	*Sine* (without)
S&S	Signs and Symptoms

S/L	Sublingual
S/P	Status Post (occurred after)
S/S	Signs and Symptoms
S1, S2, S3	Sacral Vertebrae 1, 2, 3: First, Second or Third Heart Sound
SA	Spontaneous Abortion, Sinoatrial Node SA, Surface Area, Sinoatrial
SAE	Serious Adverse Event
SAH	Subarachnoid Hemorrhage
SAL	Saline
SaO$_2$	Systemic Arterial Oxygen Saturation (%)
SARS	Severe Acute Respiratory Syndrome
SAS	Signs and Symptoms
SBE	Shortness of Breath on Exertion, Subacute Bacterial Endocarditis
SBFT	Small Bowel Follow-Through Series
SC	Subcutaneously
SCAN	Suspected Child Abuse or Neglect
SCC	Subclavian Catheter
SCD	Sequential Compression Device, Sickle Cell Disease, Sudden Cardiac Death
SCI	Spinal Cord Injury
SCICU	Spinal Cord Intensive Care Unit
SCID	Severe Combined Immunodeficiency Disease
SCLC	Small-Cell Lung Cancer
SDAT	Senile Dementia of Alzheimer's Type
SDU	Step Down Unit
Sed rate	Sedimentation Rate
SGOT	Serum Glutamic-Oxaloacetic Transaminase or Aspartate Aminotransferase
SGPT	Serum Glutamic-Pyruvic Transaminase or Alanine Aminotransferase
SH	Social History
SICU	Surgical Intensive Care Unit
SIDS	Sudden Infant Death Syndrome
sig	Instructions or Directions
SJS	Steven-Johnson Syndrome
sl	Sublingual
SLB	Short Leg Brace
SLC	Short Leg Cast

SLCC	Short Leg Cylinder Cast
SLE	Systemic Lupus Erythematosus
SLR	Straight Leg Raising
SM	Simple Mastectomy
SMA–6	Sequential Multichannel Autoanalyzer 6 (A battery of 6 tests performed on blood serum)
SMA–12	Sequential Multichannel Autoanalyzer 12 (A battery of 12 tests performed on blood serum)
SMBFT	Small Bowel Follow-Through
SMR	Submucous Resection
SniF	Subacute Nursing Facility
SO	Standing Order, or Significant Other
SOAP	Subjective, Objective, Assessment, and Plan
SOB	Shortness of Breath
SOMI	Sternal Occipital Mandibular Immobilization
Sono	Sonogram, Sonography
SOP	Standard Operating Protocol
SP or S/P	Status Post, Occurred After
spec	Specimen
SQ	Subcutaneously
SR	Sedimentation Rate
SS, S&S	Signs and Symptoms
SSE	Soap Suds Enema
SSPE	Subacute Sclerosis Panencephalitis
SSS	Sick Sinus Syndrome, Scalded Skin Syndrome
SSSS	Staphlococcal Scalded Skin Syndrome
Staph	Staphylococcus
Stat	*Statim* (at once, immediately)
STEMI	ST-Wave Elevation Myocardial Infarction
STSG	Split Thickness Skin Graft
supp	Suppository
suppos	Suppository
surg	Surgical
Sus	Substance Users
susp	Suspension
SVC	Superior Vena Cava
SVR	Systemic Vascular Resistance
SVT	Supra-Ventricular Tachycardia
SW	Stab Wound
Sx	Signs and Symptoms

SX	Sulfisoxazole, Symptoms
Sz	Seizure

T

T	Temperature, or Extent of Primary Tumor
T sect	Transverse Section
T&A	Tonsillectomy and Adenoidectomy
T&C	Type and Crossmatch
T&T	Time and Temperature
T1, T2, T3	Thoracic Vertebrae 1, 2, 3 ...
TA	Traumatic Arrest
Tab	Tablets
TAB	Typhoid-Paratyphoid A and B vaccine
TACH	Tachycardia, Tachypnea
TACHY	Tachycardia
TAE	Transarterial Embolization
TAH	Total Abdominal Hysterectomy
TAH/BSO	Total Abdominal Hysterectomy/Bilateral Salpingo-Oophorectomy
TAL	Tap and Lavage
TAM	Tamoxifen
TAT	Tetanus Antitoxin, Thematic Apperception Test
TB	Tuberculosis
tbc	Tuberculosis
TBS	To Be Scheduled
TBSA	Total Body Surface Area
tbsp	Tablespoon
Td	Adult Tetanus Toxoid and Reduced-Dose Diphtheria Toxoid
TD	Tardive Dyskinesia
TDK	Tardive Dyskinesia
TEE	Transesophageal Echocardiography
Tele	Telemetry, Telemetry Unit
TENS	Transcutaneous Electrical Nerve Stimulation
TGV	Transposition of Great Vessels
THA	Total Hip Arthroplasty
THBSO	Total Hysterectomy with Bilateral Salpingo-Oophorectomy
THP	Total Hip Prosthesis
THR	Total Hip Replacement

TIA	Transient Ischemic Attack
Tib-fib	Tibia and Fibula
TID	Three Times a Day
TIG	Tetanus-Immune Globulin
TKO	To Keep Open
TKR	Total Knee Replacement/Revision
TLC	Total Lung Capacity, Triple Lumen Catheter
TMP-SMX	Trimethoprim-Sulfamethoxazole
TNM	Tumor, Nodes, and Metastases
TOP	Termination of Pregnancy
TORCH	Types of Congenital Infections. Where T = Toxoplasmosis; O = Other; R = Rubella; C = Cytomegalic Inclusion Disease; H = Hepatitis B and Herpes
TOS	Thoracic Outlet Syndrome
Tox	Toxic, Toxicology, and Toxicologic
TPN	Total Parenteral Nutrition
TPR	Total Peripheral Resistance
Trig	Triglycerides
TRT	Testosterone Replacement Therapy
TRUS	Transrectal Ultrasonography
TSA	Total Shoulder Arthroplasty
TSH	Thyroid-Stimulating Hormone
T-spine	Thoracic Spine
TSPL	Transplant
TSR	Total Systemic Resistance
TSS	Toxic Shock Syndrome
TSSE	Toxic Shock Syndrome Exotoxin
TSST	Toxic Shock Syndrome Toxin
TT	Transferred To, Transit Time, Transthoracic, Transtracheal, Tube Thoracostomy, or Tuberculin Test, Tetanus Toxoid
TTE	Transthoracic Echocardiography
TTP	Thombotic Thrombocytopenic Purpura
TTP-HUS	Thrombotic Thrombocytopenic Pupura— Hemolytic Uremic Syndrome
TTU	Transthoracic Ultrasound
TU	Telemetry Unit
TUIP	Transurethral Incision of the Prostate
TULIP	Transurethral Ultrasound-Guided Laser-Induced Prostatectomy

TUMT	Transurethral Microwave Thermotherapy
TUNA	Transurethral Needle Ablation of the Prostate
TUR	Transurethral Resection
TURB	Transurethral Resection of Bladder
TURBT	Transurethral Resection of Bladder Tumor
TURP	Transurethral Resection of the Prostate, Transurethral Prostatectomy
TVH	Total Vaginal Hysterectomy
TVO	Telephone Voice Order
TVU	Transvaginal Ultrasound
Tx	Treatment

U

U&C	Usual and Customary
UA	Urinalysis, Unstable Angina, Umbilical Artery, Upper Airways, Upper Arm
UAO	Upper-Airway Obstruction
UAR	Upper-Airway Resistance
UB	Unna Boot, Upper Back, Urinary Bladder
UC	Ulcerative Colitis, Usual and Customary
UCHD	Usual Childhood Diseases
UCI	Unusual Childhood Illness
UCS	Unconscious
UD	Unit Dose
UDC	Usual Diseases of Childhood
UDO	Undetermined Origin
UDUN	Under-Developed Under-Nourished
UE	Upper Extremity
UES	Upper Esophageal Sphincter
UFH	Unfractionated Heparin
UGI	Upper Gastrointestinal
UGIB	Upper-Gastrointestinal Bleeding, Upper-Gastrointestinal Biopsy
UGIH	Upper-Gastrointestinal Hemorrhage
UGIS	Upper-Gastrointestinal Series
UGIS/SMFT	Upper-Gastrointestinal Series with Small Bowel Follow Through
umb	Umbilicus
UNK	Unknown
UPPP	Uvulopalatopharyngoplasty
UPT	Urinary Pregnancy Test

URI	Upper Respiratory Tract Infection, Upper Respiratory Infection
Urol	Urology
URQ	Upper-Right Quadrant
URTI	Upper Respiratory Tract Infection
US	Ultrasound
USGH	Usual State of Good Health
USH	Usual State of Health
USOGH	Usual State of Good Health
USOH	Usual State of Health
UTD	Up-to-Date
UTI	Urinary Tract Infection
UV	Ultraviolet
UVJ	Ureterovesical Junction
UVR	Ultraviolet Radiation
UWUN	Underweight Undernourished

V

V/Q	Ventilation/Perfusion (scan)
VA	Veterans Administration (a veterans administration hospital)
VAD	Vincristine, Doxorubicin and Dexamethasone.
V-Back	Vaginal Delivery after a Cesarean Section
VBG	Venous Blood Gas
VCU	Voiding Cystourethrogram
VCUG	Voiding Cystourethrogram
VD	Venereal Disease
VF	Ventricular Fibrillation, Ventricular Flutter, Visual Field, Field of Vision
VH	Vaginal Hysterectomy
VO	Verbal Order
VPC	Ventricular Premature Contractions
VS	Vital Signs
VSD	Ventriculoseptal Defect
VSS	Vital Signs Stable
VT	Tidal Volume, Ventricular Tachycardia
VTE	Venous Thromboembolism
VV	Varicose Veins
VZIG	Varicella-Zoster-Immune Globulin
VZV	Varicella-Zoster Virus

W

W/	With
W/C	Wheelchair
W/V	Weight by Volume
WBAT	Weight Bearing as Tolerated
WBC	White Blood Cell
WC	Workmans Compensation
WCC	White Cell Count
WDE	Wound Dressing Emulsion
WDWN	Well-Developed and Well-Nourished
WDWNBF	Well-Developed, Well-Nourished Black Female
WDWNBM	Well-Developed, Well-Nourished Black Male
WDWNWF	Well-Developed, Well-Nourished White Female
WDWNWM	Well-Developed, Well-Nourished White Male
WF	White Female
WM	White Male
WN	Well-Nourished
WNL	Within Normal Limits
WNV	West Nile Virus
WO, W/O	Without
WPD	Warm, Pink, and Dry
WPW	Wolff-Parkinson-White
WPWS	Wolff-Parkinson-White Syndrome
Wt	Weight
WW	White Woman

X

X	Multiplied by, Times (as in "3 × Per Day")
XIP	X-ray in Plaster
XR	X-ray
XRT	Radiation Therapy
XX	Female Sex Chromosome
XY	Male Sex Chromosome

Y

Y/O	Year Old
YAG	Yttrium-Aluminum Garnet

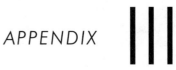

Medical Chart Checklists

PHYSICIAN OFFICE CHART CHECKLIST

- Telephone log
- E-mail log
- Narrative of office treatments
- Consultation reports
- Laboratory reports
- Radiology reports
- Vaccination log
- Executed consent for procedure forms
- Office policy and procedures relevant to incident
- Local pharmacy record

HOSPITAL CHART CHECKLIST

- Ambulance call report
- Emergency department record
- Hospital transfer record
- Preoperative testing records
- Preoperative medical clearance note
- Physician admission and progress notes
- Nurse admission and progress notes
- Physician order forms
- Laboratory reports
- Radiology reports

- Pathology report
- Consultant's reports
- Operative reports (for each operation or procedure)
- Consent for treatment forms (for each procedure)
- Pharmacy records
- Discharge summary
- Autopsy report
- Hospital policy (relevant to incident)

CLINIC CHART CHECKLIST

- Preoperative testing records
- Presurgical medical clearance note
- Physician admission and narrative treatment reports
- Nursing admission and narrative treatment reports
- Laboratory reports
- Radiology reports
- Consultant reports
- Executed consent for procedure forms
- Vaccination log
- Transfer notes to specialty clinics
- Clinic attendance log
- Pharmacy record (from the clinic or community pharmacy)
- Clinic policy and procedure (relevant to the incident case)

ASSURING A COMPLETE MEDICAL CHART

The following checklist is comprised of questions that a medical chart reviewer should ask himself or herself after having read the medical chart. If the answer to all the questions is not "yes," then the issue should be investigated further. The reviewer may have to make further requests for specific documents.

FINDING WHAT'S MISSING FROM THE MEDICAL RECORD

- Do all physician orders for radiology tests have a corresponding radiology report?
- Do all physician orders for laboratory tests have a corresponding laboratory report?
- Do all physician orders for medication have a corresponding entry in the nurse administration record?
- Do all requests for consultations in the physician order form have a corresponding consultant's report?

- Do all consultants' recommendations for action (e.g., medication, diagnostic tests, surgery, or other consultations) have a corresponding order in the physician's order form?
- Are all tests mentioned in the autopsy protocol found within the autopsy report?
- Do all nurse requests for action or evaluation have a corresponding physician note documenting findings or other actions?
- Are all incidents mentioned in physician notes also found in nursing notes?
- Are all incidents found in nursing notes also found in physician notes?

Index